Dress Scandinavian

10 9 8 7 6 5 4 3 2 1

Ebury Press, an imprint of Ebury Publishing,
20 Vauxhall Bridge Road, London, SW1V 2SA

Ebury Press is part of the Penguin Random House
group of companies whose addresses can be found
at global.penguinrandomhouse.com

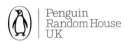

Penguin
Random House
UK

Copyright © Pernille Teisbæk, 2017
Photography © Oscar Meyer, Nicolaj Didriksen
and private photos, 2017

Pernille Teisbæk has asserted her right to be
identified as the author of this Work in accordance
with the Copyright, Designs and Patents Act 1988

Originally published in Danish by The People's Press, 2016

First published by Ebury Press in 2017

www.penguin.co.uk

A CIP catalogue record for this book is available
from the British Library

Redesign for UK edition by Imagist, original design by LOW Studios

ISBN: 9781785037061

Printed and bound in Italy by L.E.G.O. S.p.A.

Penguin Random House is committed to a
sustainable future for our business, our readers
and our planet. This book is made from Forest
Stewardship Council® certified paper.

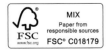

MIX
Paper from
responsible sources
FSC® C018179
FSC
www.fsc.org

Dress Scandinavian

Pernille Teisbæk

EBURY
PRESS

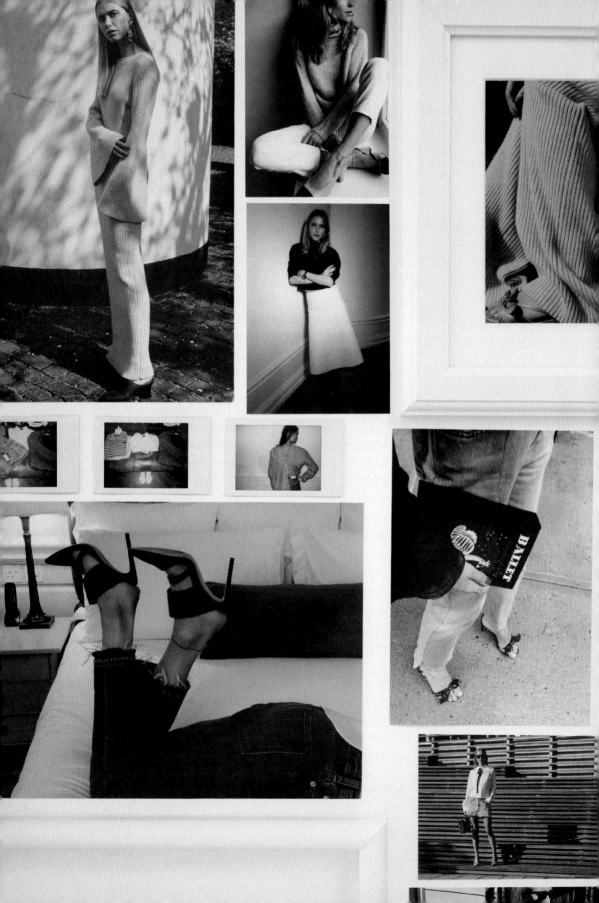

Introduction

Within the world of fashion, Scandinavian design has obtained a rather remarkable position. It's a style that signals confidence and self-assurance – and rightfully so. There is indeed much to be proud of, and Scandinavian fashion has a lot to offer in terms of inspiration. In truth, most people are partial to comfortable clothes and Scandinavian fashion is quite simple and easy to wear. Comfort radiates confidence and strength. Naturally, this does not mean that the Scandinavian wardrobe consists of only soft Kashmir leisure suits and ergonomic trainers. On the contrary, we maintain a delicate balance between current fashions and our own personal style. Easier said than done, I know. Which is why I wish to share my ideas on how to create a great basic wardrobe, the 'do's and don'ts' of Scandinavian fashion. I will also share personal experiences from my life, as they have taught me a lot, and hopefully my experiences will inspire you.

First of all, I would like to introduce three guidelines that are useful in my work as a stylist and in my private life, regardless of whether I'm deciding what to wear or what to buy.

A simple outfit does not necessarily equal a boring outfit. In fact, it can often have the exact opposite effect in the eye of the beholder. If you decide to mix just a few styles and you combine them in a completely personal way for example an exquisite shirt with a pair of jeans and high heels, this can be very effective. We are not talking about a revolutionary look, but rather a classic outfit that makes you feel comfortable. There is no need for camouflage in the shape of a jacket and you don't need to upgrade with lots of accessories. The noisier your outfit, the more it craves attention, which is not always preferable. Focus on the small details in your 'less-is-more' look, as this will help you to ensure that it is indeed spot-on – read more about this in chapter 2.

Less is more

Quality does not equal expensive designer brands. Personally, I wear a lot of high-street fashion, as they too manage the exquisite timeless designs that you can use season after season. Invest in that one pair of perfect-fitting jeans rather than buying three pairs that only fit you so-so. It's not about wearing a new pair of jeans every day, it's about getting that one pair that works for you, which you can then combine with other clothes and accessories to continue to create new looks for yourself.

Quality vs. Quantity

We all have clothes' crises, not least each time the seasons change and we have to reinvent our wardrobe. The best piece of advice I can give you in those situations is to get a good overview of what you actually have in your wardrobes – and then get rid of every single item that you no longer use. This will help you avoid having to decide between five cream-coloured tops. One always fits you better than the rest; something we often tend to forget. So take the time to go through everything you own and don't be afraid to get rid of stuff, as this will give you a much better starting point and you won't have to spend time trying on numerous styles that are basically identical.

When I attend fashion weeks or meet people through work, I always sense their excitement when I tell them where I'm from. Why is that? It's not like we're comparable to the chic Parisiennes, who always manage the perfect 'I've-just-got-out-of-bed-but-I-still-look-like-a-million -dollars' look, or the boho-chic-LA look, which is both raw and feminine and never goes out of fashion.

I believe that our uniqueness and our ability to excite others stems from the way we combine colours and materials and from our urge to create new silhouettes, which focus on minimalism and comfort. A great example is the Thai fisherman's trousers; a pair of oversized trousers with no zip, elastic band or buttons, where you use a special folding technique to tie them together. They are one size only and originally from Thailand, but they made it all the way to Scandinavia on account of being extremely comfortable. The trend for an oversized dress / T-shirt worn with matching tight leggings or jeans is similarly comfortable.

Our outfits do not ooze sex appeal; in fact, they are rather androgynous, though never completely masculine. It's a look that suits our natural make-up as well as our full eyebrows and hair, which provides us with an organic and healthy finish.

More than anything, our strength lies in being able to create a look that is timeless without being boring, where we use old classics but style them in a contemporary and effortless manner. Examples include wearing a casual hoodie under a stylish black blazer, or using a scarf as a belt in your Levi's 501's. It's not about investing in lots of expensive items; it's about personalizing each item and reusing them over and over again, but in new ways.

The Scandinavian style changes over time, as does every other style, but there are some fundamental reasons why it is minimalistic. I personally believe that it stems from our reluctance to stand out; instead we express ourselves in the details. I see a strong link between the communal who-do-you-think-you-are attitude (the Law of Jante) and our collective way of dressing. To an outsider, it's rather obvious that most Danish people dress in a similar way, with the exception of small details. Initially, this may appear quite inspiring, but once you have spent some time in Denmark, it becomes rather less exciting. On the other hand, Scandinavians, when compared to the rest of Europe, are quite independent and confident. We leave home at an early age, many of us work from a young age to make some pocket money, and we are keen to take care of ourselves from early on. And perhaps our clothes simply reflect that we actively choose to look alike; that we want to share our confidence.

I believe that it's always a good idea to travel, be it to big cities or more rural areas, to observe the variations presented in local streetscapes, as this will help you develop your own personal style. Sit down at an outdoor café and allow your eyes to wander. Take your time. Observe the old as well as the young. A printed scarf may catch your eye, or a cool hat, or even just a colourful sock sticking out from a shoe. In my opinion, it is something we do well, allowing ourselves to be inspired. I travel to gain inspiration from foreign styles, and I always learn something new. Remember that it's okay to stand out from the masses, to challenge oneself, to become a frontrunner with some small detail, while still remaining within your comfort zone.

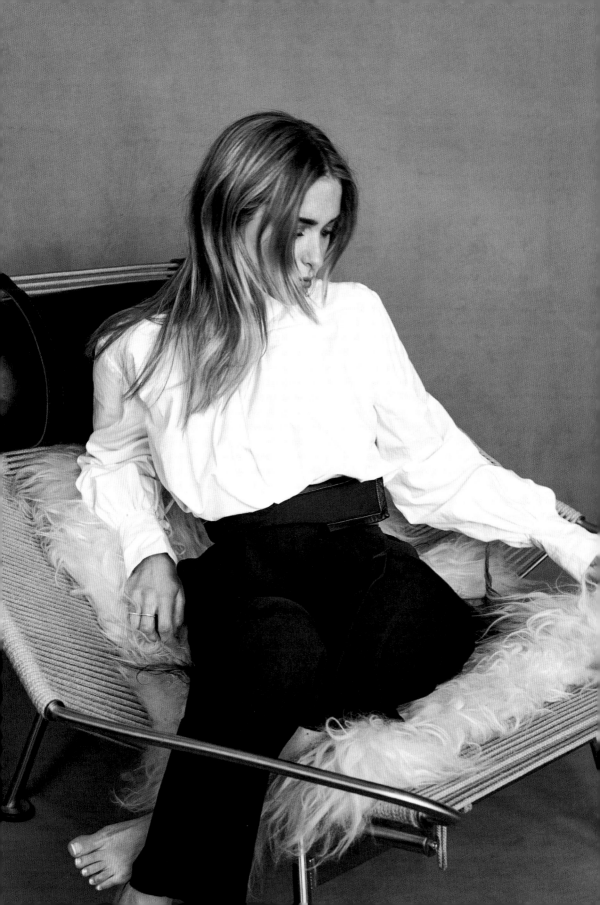

Growing Up

I've been interested in fashion for as long as I can remember. I have vivid recollections of being 10 years old, working furiously at my first sewing machine, which I inherited from my maternal grandmother. It kick-started my interest in and my knowledge about fabric, shapes and details. I quickly learnt how to combine materials and customise a classic pair of Levi's 501's.

As I grew older, I started modelling. It was a great student job and a welcome break from school. It gave me new insights into the world of fashion, not least because I would see the collections before they became available to the general public. Being so closely involved with a fashion house where I got to see the love that designers have for their designs, and their dedication, was hugely inspiring to me. However, I quickly found what I really liked doing: styling. I always had an opinion about what I was wearing – which was probably frustrating for the stylists working with me! – but it would eventually prove to be my gateway into the world of fashion. I was doing a cover shoot for *WOMAN*, the first magazine I worked for, when I came up with an idea for my look. They readily accepted it, even if styling was not really part of a model's job description. Soon after, the fashion editor of the magazine encouraged me to apply for her position, as she had just resigned. I applied for the job without batting an eyelid, despite not knowing what it actually entailed! Fortunately I got the job, and my time as a fashion editor definitely helped widen my knowledge of the many areas that make up the world of fashion; in front of, but also behind, the camera.

When I was starting out as a fashion editor, I was also studying design technology, which meant juggling quite a lot at the same time! I was managing weekly deadlines for a fashion series, guides, articles and cover shoots while simultaneously finishing the education that helped me to develop my knowledge of design and learn more about the great (and not so great) aspects of the fashion industry. Having the opportunity to inspire other people with my knowledge and personal taste is a privilege, and the next obvious step for me was starting my blog, 'LookdePernille'.

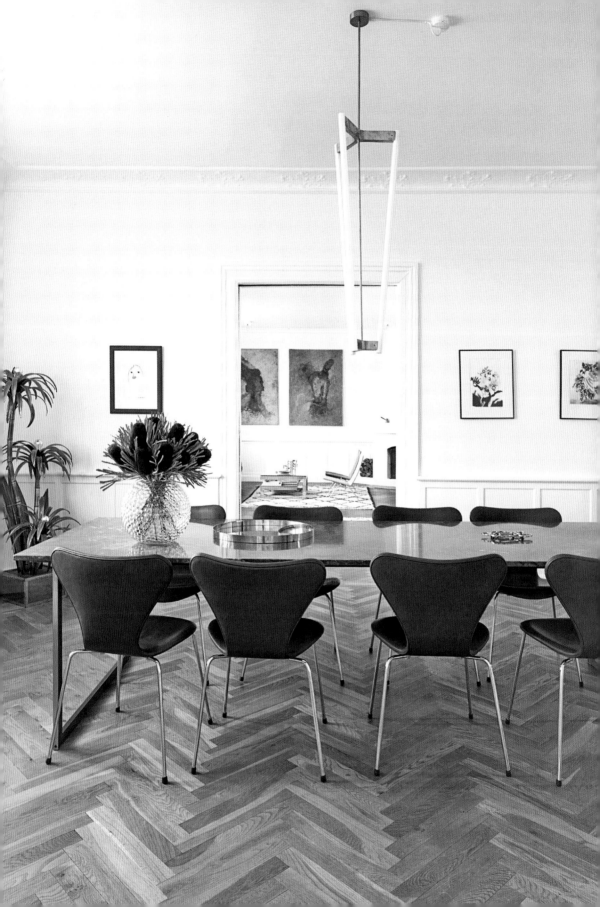

My area of expertise soon became Scandinavian style, something I love working with for lots of different reasons. Scandinavian classics not only influence the way I dress but my entire home. It's obviously an investment that takes time as well as money, but to me fashion, art, architecture and design are all interconnected. The combination of streamlined and organic shapes, lots of personality and exciting materials create the framework for the ultimate Scandinavian home. For example, when you mix leather, wood, metal and stone in the design of your home, it makes for something truly unique. Up until a few years ago, I spent most of my money on clothes. But when I turned 30, which felt both frightening but also the beginning of a new era, I decided that my birthday present to myself would be a piece of furniture, which would last my lifetime. It was an investment that left no money for clothes, but I've never regretted it as for many years I'd been in love with Wegner's Flag Halyard chair, a simple chair that combines various materials in a wonderful way.

It was the beginning of a new interest, which is slowly taking up more and more of my time. As much as I like to dress well, I also like being surrounded by nice things. I love travelling, but I also find great pleasure in staying at home. It's important to have a 'safe haven' where you're surrounded by gorgeous items that you really care about.

In Scandinavia, we spend more time in our homes than almost anywhere else in the world. Which is why it makes sense that we create some of the world's most spectacular houses. We personalise our homes and we pay a lot of attention to detail. I grew up surrounded by classic furniture by masters such as Arne Jacobsen, Finn Juhl and Børge Mogensen without even realising, but it definitely helped shape my aesthetic palette. It's funny to think about how the furniture in my home from 20 years ago has only improved with age, benefitting from the patina that comes with experiencing life.

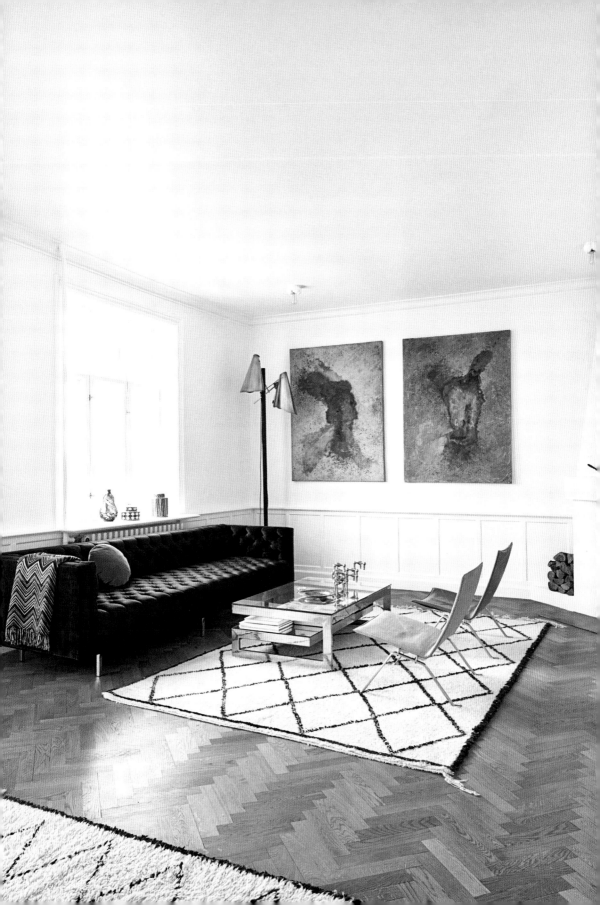

In Denmark, we often talk about 'hygge' ('cosiness' for lack of a better translation), about the importance of creating a cosy and comfortable home. 'Hygge' has been discussed a lot recently, as people around the world have become interested in this Danish concept, which, at its heart, encompasses every emotion related to wellbeing. It's a word we also use to describe the way we dress, but oddly enough, it's not a word that's easily translated into other languages. There are a lot of similarities I have found between the way we dress and the way we like to design our homes:

1 Minimalism: we always prefer simple colours and streamlined shapes.

2 Personality: we love to incorporate an unexpected detail. This could be something like a colourful scarf or maybe a framed poster from a flea market.

3 Mixed materials: whether it's cotton and lacquer or metal and leather, we like to combine different elements.

4 Comfort and 'hygge': this is always a high priority, which makes us the world's happiest people!

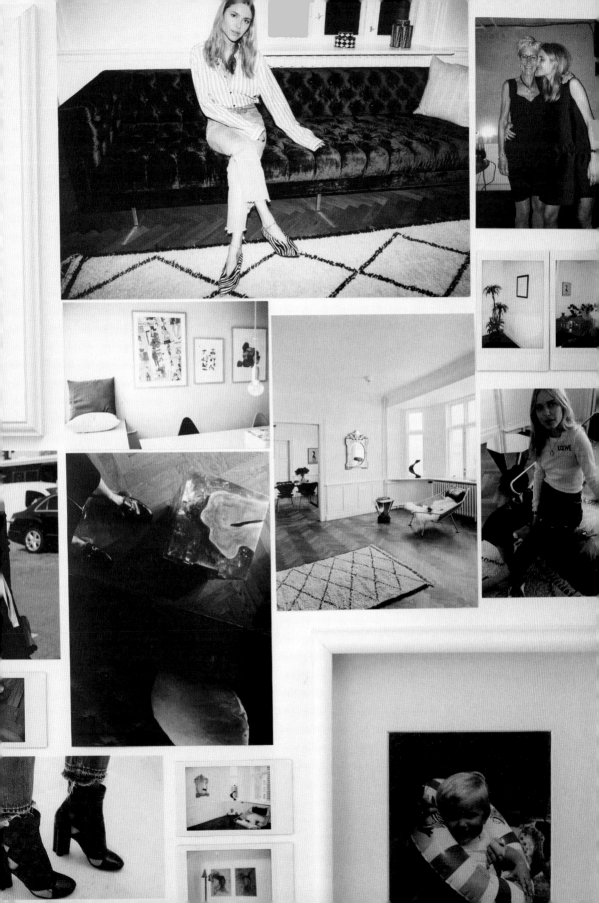

It's All in the Details

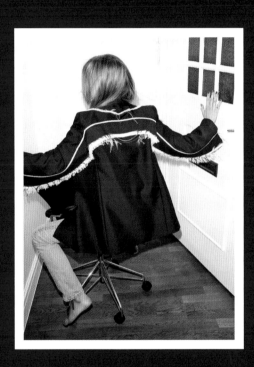

Twice a year, I go on what I think of as a 'tour de fashion week'. This usually starts in Berlin, and from there I go on to Copenhagen, Stockholm, New York, London, Milan and finally Paris. It usually takes about a-month-and-a-half, and I'm completely worn out when it's over! Several of my friends, and not least my family, can't understand why I force myself to complete this fashion marathon, when I could simply stream shows at Vogue.com or look at the millions of photos posted on Instagram. But this is because they don't know any better! Yes, I *could* watch the shows on the Internet, but then I'd miss out on the atmosphere, the set designs and the music specifically chosen to underpin the feeling each designer wants to convey to their audience as we watch their collections. And I wouldn't get that tangible experience of seeing the different materials combined in various ways live. Watching shows online also makes it difficult to catch the quirky details, which are so crucial to any collection. And yes, I know, we're getting a little technical here, but this is the nerd in me, so bear with me, and I'll explain exactly what I mean…

To me, an interesting detail is anything from an outer seam on a jacket to unfinished hems, a bow in a model's hair, a particular hood, a loafer, an open back or an unusual combination of materials. These details simply vanish or remain unnoticed when you watch catwalk footage, as it usually consists only of frontal shots. But it's the tiny details that update the good old classics such as a white shirt, a trench coat or a pair of jeans. It's usually also the tiny details that save us from having to go out and invest in lots of new items when wearing what you already have in a new way will often do the trick. For example, you can cut the bottom off a pair of favourite jeans and create an unfinished-hem look like the most popular jeans from Vetements as seen on Instagram. Or you can wear your shirt back-to-front, with the buttons on the back, which gives you a low-cut back and a high collar in front much like J. W. Anderson's shirts. These are details we can all afford and they immediately update your look significantly.

I love the beginning of a new season, and I love noticing the unusual things that may escape others. However, I don't just find inspiration at the big glossy fashion shows. I'm really inspired by streetscapes, and also how each city uses catwalk pieces to reflect its own style. It feels like they grow increasingly wild from one year to the next. It's fun to watch how fashion is adapted in each location.

Use a printed scarf rather than a regular belt and tie it in a small knot at the side of your jeans or trousers. This can really lift a look from being just average to personal and fun.

Wear a satin ribbon tied in a bow with your shirt in place of a tie – it's an easy and elegant upgrade for an evening out.

Wear your sandals with a glittery sock in winter.

Get much more use out of your fancy dresses by wearing them over trousers; it's a great casual contrast to an otherwise dressed-up look.

Spruce up any weekday outfit of old jeans and a T-shirt with an eye-catching pair of red high heels.

I have no wish to change my style each season in order to keep up with current fashion trends. I prefer to do it my way, which means playing around with details. In fact, I consider my wardrobe a dressing-up treasure trove, where I try things out on myself before using them in a campaign or a fashion series.

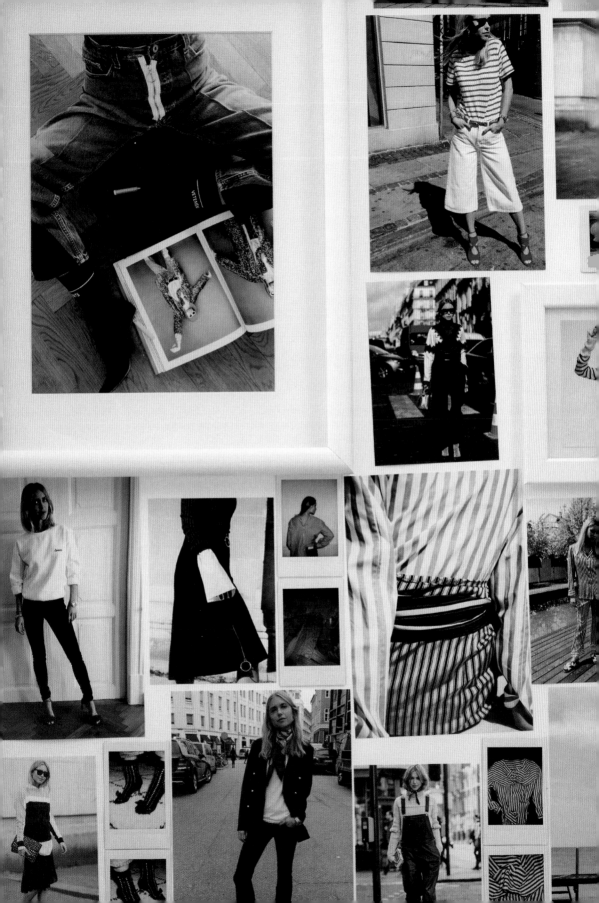

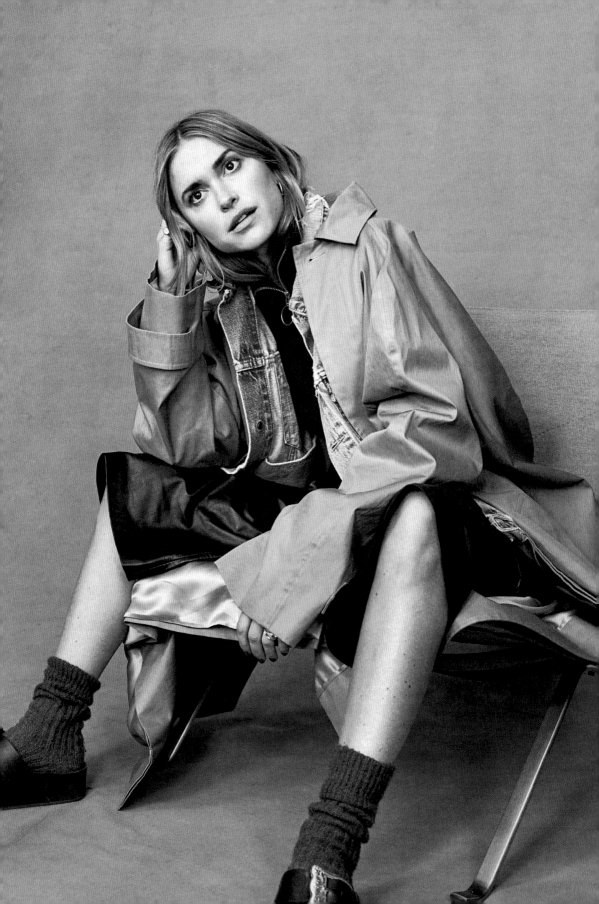

The

Androgynous

Look

Most people think of Scandinavian style as being rather minimalistic and quite androgynous. That is true, and on the surface of it that may not sound particularly appealing, but it's not to say that Scandinavians aren't feminine. Several of the essential styles in any Scandinavian basic wardrobe are definitely unisex, and sometimes your entire outfit might belong to your partner, brother, father or male friend! There is a good reason for this, though. A masculine shape will accentuate feminine features. If, for instance, you wear a broad-shouldered blazer with a simple tank top and a pair of tight-fitting jeans, your figure will immediately appear quite petite and delicate.

Coco Chanel was among the first to include the androgynous style in her wardrobe, insisting that women should not solely wear dresses. As with everything else, it's all about striking a balance, and it's important to remember that contrasts have the power to both lift and tone down any given look. A pair of men's trousers with high heels equals a lift, as your legs appear elongated and it will emphasise your feminine posture. Conversely, you can tone down a miniskirt by wearing it with a man's T-shirt or a knitted jumper, as this will diminish the sexy look and make it more casual. Both of these examples show how you can use contrasts to create different and exciting looks.

The White Shirt

It's a cliché, I know, that we all have to have a white shirt in our wardrobe. But it's also true, because it's important to have great basic styles that you can use again and again, without anyone noticing. And that makes the white shirt your best friend. You can easily style a white shirt in various ways without losing its classic appeal. It allows you to express your personality, as it's not a focus-grabber, and it leaves your face and body a 'blank canvas'. It's certainly not revolutionary in any way, but each new season presents a new opportunity of what it should and could look like. I have often worn the same jeans for a whole week (really!), only I've styled them in different ways, which meant that nobody noticed – or at least nobody said anything!

If you ask me, you should always buy the most simple white shirt. It doesn't have to be an expensive shirt, but it should always be good quality, otherwise it may shrink or become grey when washed. The main thing is that it should fit perfectly across both shoulders and your bosom. Of course, you can always buy more shirts with a different cut or varying details. Just be careful not to overdo it though, as it will only generate more confusion; trust me.

Personally, I always have the same two shirts in my wardrobe, which I occasionally exchange for new versions that are exactly the same, for example when there are a few too many red wine stains that won't come out in the wash (even if I follow my mother's great advice to always leave the shirt soaking in warm water and chlorine overnight!). One shirt is a standard non-fitted white shirt with a regular collar and lapels, which practically crackles once it's been ironed. The other shirt is soft and more transparent with a Mandarin collar, which goes brilliantly with a polo neck. I always bring one or the other when I'm travelling because I can wear them with practically everything.

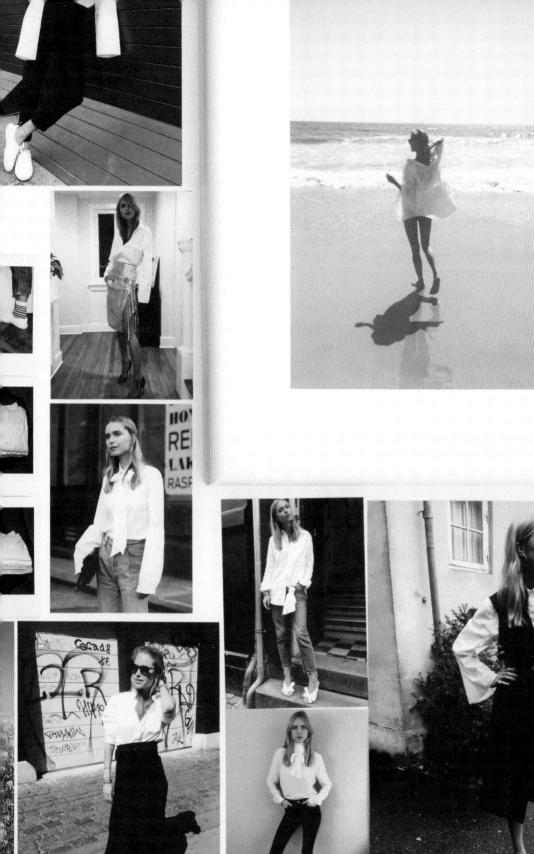

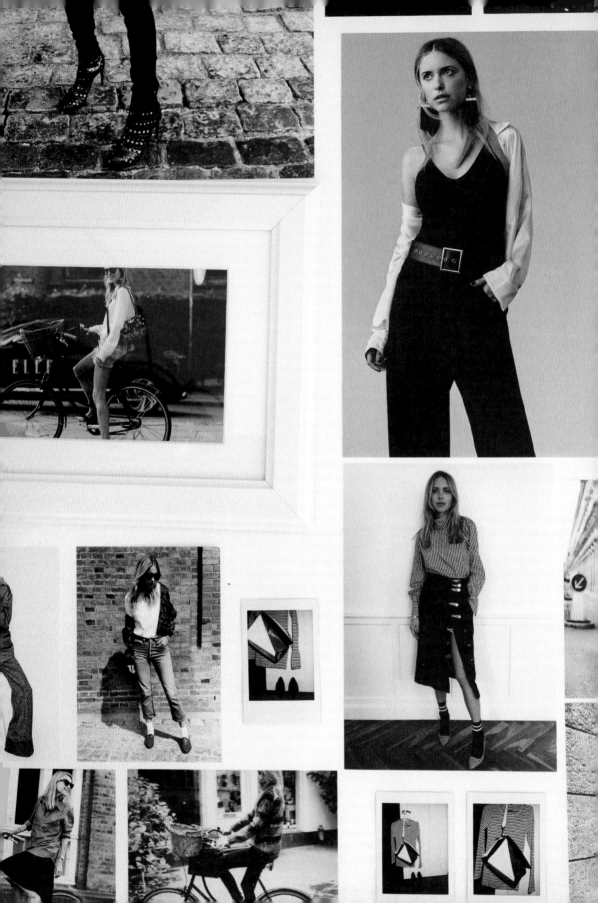

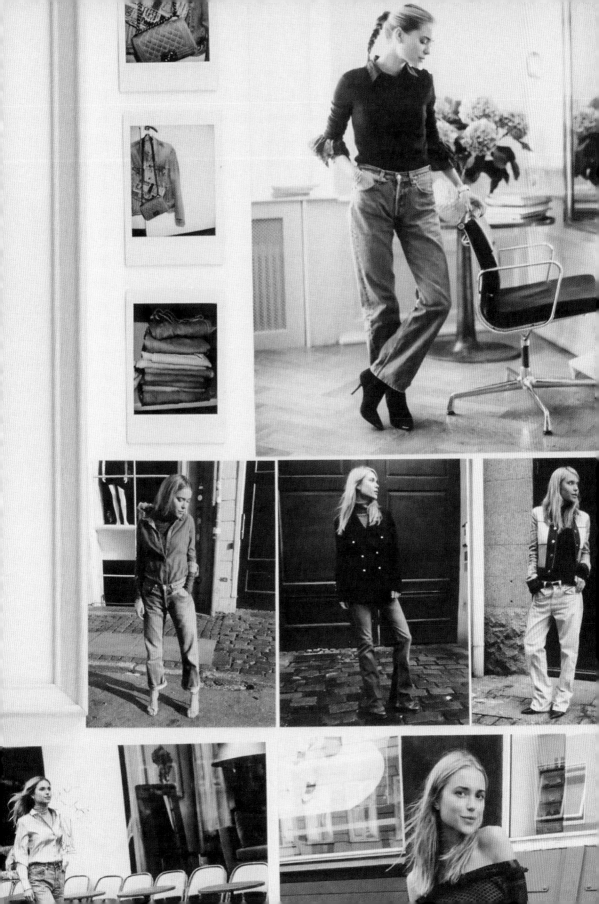

Jeans
(and which shape fits which body)

Jeans are one of my favourite items of clothing, and I'll happily wear the same pair again and again. I know that a lot of people find buying jeans stressful, which is why many decide to simply not purchase them, as they can't face the ordeal of trying on numerous pairs until they find the one that fits!

So, lesson number one is to completely disregard what sales assistants or fashion magazines claim to be trending at the time. Instead, focus on finding the right jeans for your body shape. Furthermore, never buy jeans online, unless you've already tried them on and know exactly which size to buy. There's also a big difference between untreated denim and pre-washed. My jeans size vary from brand to brand, which can be really annoying, especially if you can't always be bothered to try them on when you're in the shop.

People have different opinions about whether its best to buy expensive or cheap jeans. However, it's important to keep in mind that high prices do not guarantee a better fit or durability. I, for one, should definitely be more selective when it comes to jeans. I have to admit to having pairs I no longer wear! My collection of jeans is a wonderful mix of high-street brands, second-hand jeans and some rather exclusive jeans, but my favourite pair cost only 10 pounds. I still can't bring myself to throw them out, despite the fact that they now have numerous patches inside and they're coming apart in critical areas, which makes wearing them quite a gamble these days! They're a pair of vintage Levi's; their boyish look is not terribly flattering and they most definitely fall under the androgynous category, but they are incredibly comfortable, which is a criteria not to be underestimated.

There are lots of different styles of jeans, and here I've described a few of my favourites. But once again, I'd like to stress that the only things that really matter are body shape and comfort. So please do not regard this as a 'jeans-bible'; it's no more than a list based on my experiences, which may hopefully provide a little guidance as you try to discover your own personal favourites.

'Boyfriend' jeans are my all-time favourite fit. Comfortable, yet rough and androgynous, their anti-fit adds volume to an already wonderfully curved bottom, which is why it's important to combine them with something tight-fitting on top.

The jeans should hang from your hip, which may shorten your legs, but that's nothing a pair of high heels can't fix for those of us who weren't born with long legs. Short trouser legs reveal slender ankles, and if you want to use them in winter simply add a pair of glittery socks, and you're good to go.

Boyfriend

The 1970s and flared jeans certainly left their mark on the denim world, and this extremely flattering fit has been a hit ever since. Boho-chic women have embraced the look because flared jeans accentuate feminine curves and even create shape for those who are not so curvy. If your legs are short, flared jeans will help you 'hide' a platform shoe, making your legs look longer. If you don't want to wear high platform shoes, try high-waisted jeans instead.

However avoid the high-cut waist if you have a slightly wider waist; you should go for a low-cut waist and boot-cut leg, which is a little less flared but still gives you that sexy and curvy figure.

If you'd asked me less than two years ago, Mom jeans would have been on the list of things I wouldn't be seen dead in – so what happened?

Well, I'd better explain what Mom jeans are, in case you don't know. Mom jeans are high-waisted jeans that fit you in all the wrong places. And yet Mom jeans will shape you in ways you never thought possible. People with a Beyoncé booty will love them, as they include 100 per cent 'bum-benefits'. However, if, like myself, you don't have the singularly female curves, your bum will appear rather dull and flat because the pockets are placed a little higher than usual. Which is why I've tended to avoid them. On the other hand, the high waist is extremely comfortable (once you get used to it) and it defines your waist while concealing any love handles. Within the last couple of years, comfort has become increasingly important to me. I no longer suffer for beauty, so lo and behold, my wardrobe now includes a pair of Mom jeans! My first purchase in this style was a pair of vintage jeans, which proved a soft transition to the coarser version from Vetements, which is now on my top three list.

Slim Fit

It's not a diet formula, but it is undoubtedly the most flattering jeans style. It's tight around your legs with a little extra room around the front pockets and along the groin. My personal favourites are the low-waisted styles with a slightly higher back, which gives your bottom a really great shape. This is also the style I most frequently use with my layer-on-layer look (which you can read more about in Chapter 6). This style is perfect for muscular legs because it elongates them – even when you're wearing trainers. Everyday heels will work wonders for your behind and really accentuate a feminine posture.

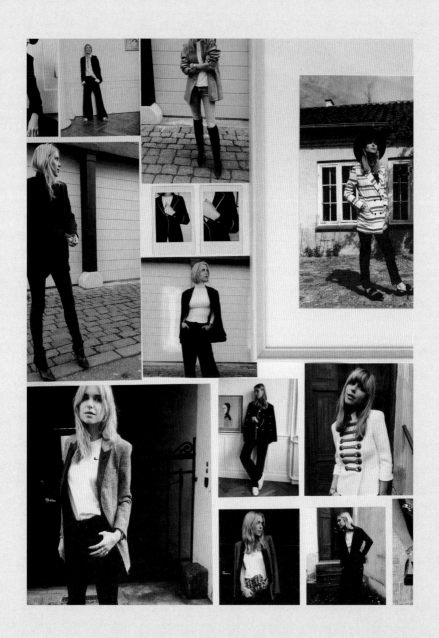

Blazer

A short blazer goes really well with a dress, high-waisted skirt or trousers, as it will highlight your feminine shape.

A long blazer works well with low-waisted jeans and a blouse, transforming it into a casual suit.

An oversized blazer provides a perfect masculine contrast to a simple and understated look. It's also ideal for layering, worn with a hoodie or chunky knitwear underneath.

The blazer is indispensable if you ask me, as it will instantly upgrade even a really dull outfit. I often wear a blazer instead of a coat or jacket when I'm sporting my layer-on-layer look. It's important to get a multi-purpose blazer as it can also make a more classic look feel more casual.

I vividly remember buying my first blazer – it was silk-satin with no lining and it had more of a cardigan feel than anything, which suited my less formal taste in those days. Since then, I've owned lots of different styles of blazer. The cut is absolutely crucial in terms of comfort, and it pays to invest in a high-quality woollen blazer with satin lining, as it will last longer.

So, should you go for a long or short version, a square or fitted version? Well, it's important that you don't buy the first classic blazer you come across as it may well be too broad across the shoulders and too long; instead think about what would best suit your figure. It's important not to compromise on the fit – the shoulders and the sleeves should fit you perfectly.

It's also worth paying attention to the lapel when deciding on your personal, perfect blazer. The lapel can vary in size as well as shape and it determines how low-cut the front will appear. You should also consider whether you'd like side or back slits, as they will help you move more freely and make sure you can rummage through your trouser pockets! Most fashion houses have removed this little detail, which is an indication of looks over comfort. And speaking of details; if your blazer has side pockets then make sure you never use them, as this will only make them sag and droop.

Trainers

We've all been there, waking up in the morning and slipping into comfortable everyday clothes, but then you face a tough decision: heels or trainers? A few years ago, my automatic reply would have been heels, but lately, I've become quite fond of comfy shoes, exactly because they are extremely comfortable and you can wear them with anything from a skirt to jeans; at home or at work. Flat shoes have gained permanent residency in the Scandinavian wardrobe, including mine. I'll even quite happily don a pair of trainers for a special occasion, whereas previously I would have always worn heels.

Although I'm a huge fan of American culture, I won't wear any old trainers. I'm a strong believer in the simple, preppy tennis style such as the Superga. Their look is unisex, clean and classic. Which is also why they go so well with the androgynous look. The Nike trainer has also become a more-or-less permanent fixture on more sporty types. Scandinavians definitely value comfortable footwear – and I guess there's no need to mention the numerous cobbled streets we have to walk up and down!

Today, the flat trainer is for everybody, whether you prefer a 1990s vintage trainer like the Nike Air Max that comes in every colour, or you are a true collector sporting a pair of exclusive Yeezy Boost created by Adidas in collaboration with Kanye West. The expensive trainers have taken this otherwise low-key trend to completely new levels, where even high-end brands like Céline and Chanel offer their take on a flat trainer.

However, wearing a pair of sneakers means you need to add some feminine details to your ensemble if you want to avoid a look that's a little *too* casual. For example, wear plain-coloured trainers with an otherwise colourful bohemian outfit to add a sporty edge to your feminine look. Or, more colourful trainers provide a great contrast to a minimalist style, adding a touch of freshness and originality. My shoe collection (which consists mainly of high heels) includes only a few pairs of black shoes while the rest are colourful.

If you don't feel it's right to wear trainers with your work outfit, below you'll find a few ground rules on how to make the most of your comfy shoes:

Trainers are supposed to be worn, so don't be afraid to get them dirty.

However, if you wear trainers to work and need to be a little smarter, bring a cloth and wipe them clean before your next meeting.

Scandinavians are great fans of wearing running shoes with everyday outfits, but trainers don't belong in a very formal office environment.

Trainers and socks are a classic combination, so make a point of matching up striking combos.

Even though jeans and trainers are a perfect match, don't forget skirts and dresses, as they can be pretty cool with a pair of kicks.

While white trainers are a sure winner, the more colourful versions can add a little spice and life to your minimalist look.

If you love the latest trainers trend, go for it! But don't be afraid to let some shoe trends pass you by, sometimes it's better to stick with your personal favourites.

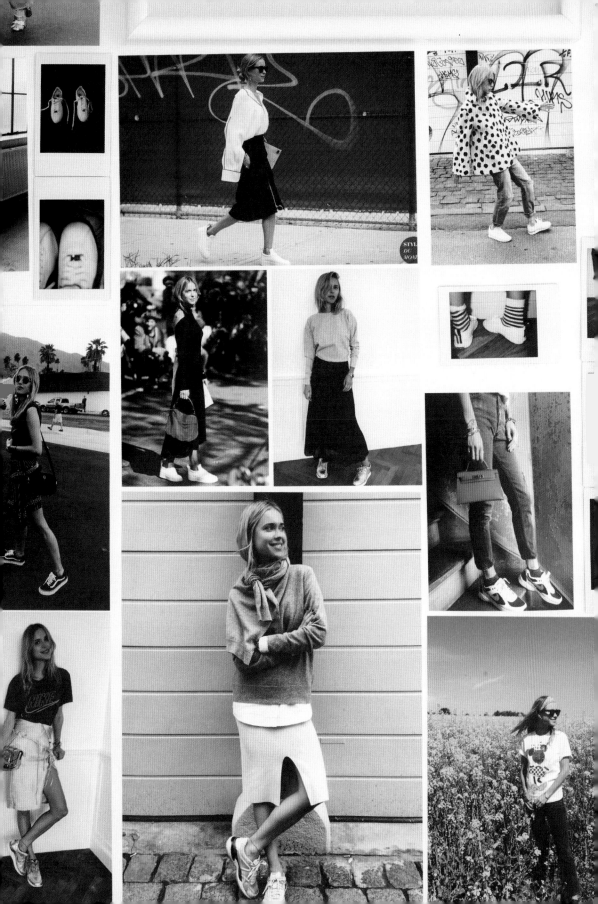

STYLE
DU
MONDE

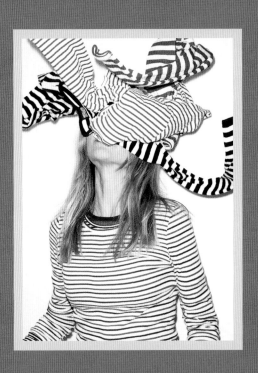

Say
it
with
stripes

Stripes are no longer uniquely French, even if Coco Chanel was the first to popularise those iconic Breton stripes. You can also see this ever-popular maritime trend in Danish fashion; although our days as a great seafaring nation are long gone, the stripes remain. Maritime stripes are a Scandinavian favourite and we happily wear both the knitted naval sweater from S.N.S. Herning and the iconic Comme des Garçons tops. The classic #101 T-shirt from Nørgaard is always a safe bet when opting for the stripy look, even if the stripes are horizontal, which is usually less flattering. Ever since Jørgen Nørgaard designed this long-sleeved T-shirt back in 1967, more than three million have been sold, and it's now considered a Danish icon. The 101s are even still produced in Denmark, which is rare these days.

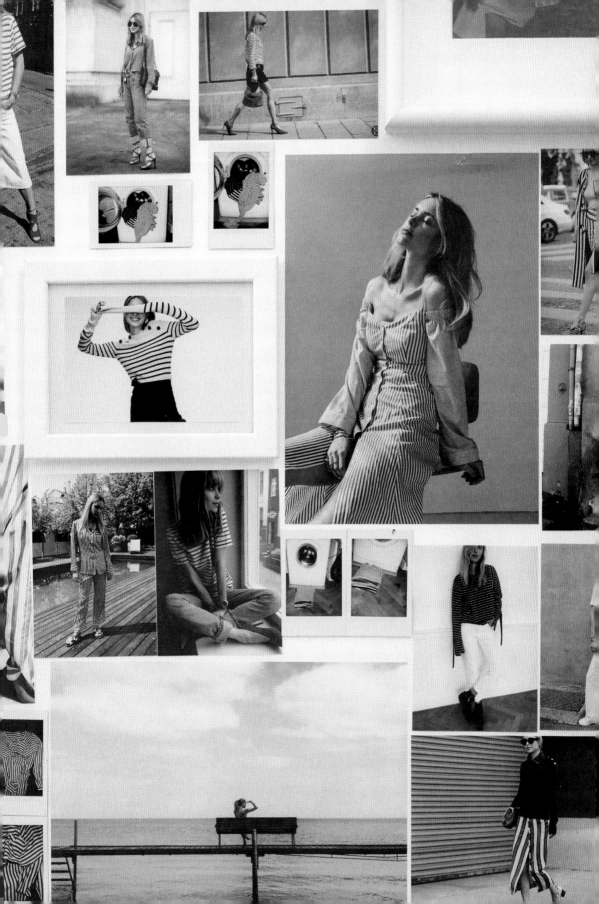

Strike a Stripe

Prints are not the first thing that spring to mind when you
think of Scandinavian design, especially if you compare us
to the more colourful Italian women, for example, who will
combine various prints in lots of different ways. When it
comes to classic stripes, though, we are second to none. We
make them work in a number of ways with our Scandinavian
monochrome look, and we combine them with new and old
classics. We might wear a striped top with a formal blazer,
where the top immediately adds a striking quality. Or we
might combine a striped top with a colourful fur coat from
Danish favourites Saks Potts, which immediately draws the
look in a more classical direction. Stripes can be used in many
and varied ways. Depending on the colour combinations,
they can be viewed as a fairly staple element in your basic
wardrobe. Thin maritime stripes on top are easily mixed
with broader stripes below, as long as you stay within similar
colour tones or go for the monochrome look. Horizontal
stripes may enhance your bosom, as they are rarely considered
slimming, but then again; whoever said they should be.

The great thing about stripes is their ability to enhance your figure when used correctly. A pair of trousers with vertical stripes will work to elongate your legs, especially if you wear them with a pair of really high heels. If you have broad shoulders and slim hips, you should opt for vertical stripes on top and horizontal stripes below – and vice-versa, if you have drooping shoulders and wide hips. You can also use small stripy details to make a difference to your overall look, for example a belt with vertical stripes will minimise your waist. Or you could wear a pair of vertically striped socks, as this will make your ankles appear slim.

The

Scandi

Colour
Palette

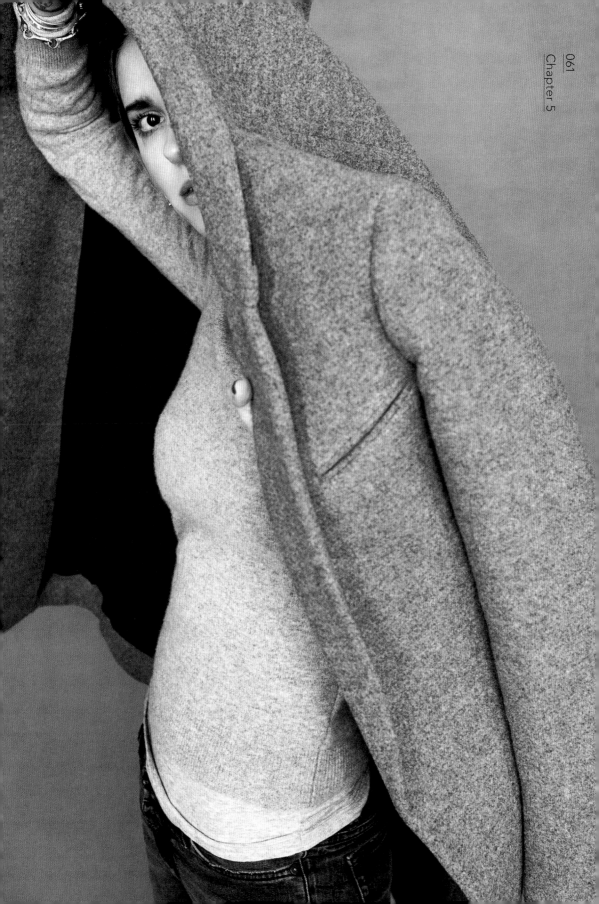

It's no secret that only a few Scandinavians wear all the colours of the rainbow. We tend to prefer more basic colours such as black, blue, grey and white as well as earthy, natural tones. From time to time, we may go wild and wear something bright red. It's not that we're afraid of colours, but naturally our fresh skin tone and blonde hair influence our colour schemes. Add to that our reluctance to stand out, and most of us end up experimenting only by combining slightly different versions of the same basic colours. However, when it comes to accessories – be it shoes or handbags – we will gladly add a touch of colour! We also often add more muted, natural colours to our otherwise monochrome layer-on-layer look. For example, wearing a pink shirt with a pair of jeans and a grey sweater means the cuffs and collar will add a splash of colour, as well as adding an interesting detail to two otherwise timeless items. The most important thing, however, is to make sure that your basic wardrobe is not lacking any key items, as this makes it much easier to add colour.

For Scandinavians though, it's not always all about colour. Just as important for us is an ability to mix materials. For example, an outfit that combines leather, denim and knitwear in the same colour is easily more exciting to us than an outfit that uses lots of different bright colours.

You won't find many colours in my wardrobe, except for a hint of red and cobalt – which incidentally go really well together! I did allow myself to buy a striped knitted sweater from Alessandro Michele's SS16 collection for Gucci, which is possibly the most colourful item I own. What I love the most about it is its perfect tones of red and blue. In some ways, you could say that this knitted sweater is timeless, both in terms of stripes and shape, yet it still manages to make even the dullest of jackets or the blandest pair of trousers feel fresh and contemporary.

Which colours go with your skin tone is utterly individual. There are no rules. But if you make your way to the chapter on Hotline Bling, you can find out how to determine whether your skin tone is cold or warm on page 99. Keep in mind that the chapter is merely a guideline – we should all get to know which colours add life and glow to our face, and which ones bring out the dark rings under our eyes or drain our skin. Plus, remember to test your skin tone in daylight rather than electric light.

If You Have a Cold Skin Tone...

You should wear cold and strong colours; those with an underlying blue hue. Obvious choices are black, white, light grey, charcoal grey, ice-blue and blue-black – picture a cold, frosty winter's day. However, practically all colours are available in a cold version, even mustard yellow and red.

If You Have a Warm Skin Tone...

You should wear softer, earthy colours with yellow or golden undertones. Picture autumn leaves and charred colours such as red, saturated yellow, bottle-green and a warm brown. But again, even the coldest colours have warm siblings, including cobalt, marine and reddish-purple.

Choosing colours that complement your skin tone is a great rule of thumb, which has been in use for decades, and it's very useful when you find yourself looking for new clothes or when you end up in that same old dilemma of having to choose between two dresses. However, whatever your skin tone, you can still wear colours that are not part of your basic palette, as long as you don't overdo it – maybe only go full throttle with your accessories. You should always avoid wearing colours that don't work well for your skin tone right up against your face though, as they are likely to make you look ill. If you want to wear such colours on your torso, make sure you soften it with a colour that's a perfect match for you, for example, by adding a scarf or revealing a shirt collar.

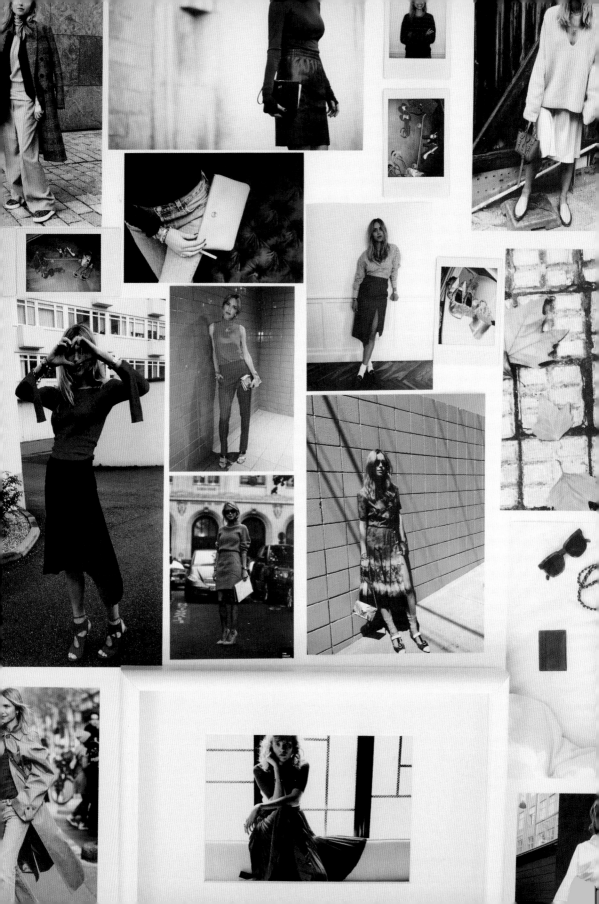

Complementary colour combinations, do just that: they complement each other. It's the merging of opposites, which I often use in my work as a stylist. Red and green, yellow and purple as well as blue and orange are typical complementary colours. You don't necessarily have to choose 'pure' combinations; you can also use various nuances such as navy blue and gold, Bordeaux-red and bottle-greens or camel and Bordeaux-red.

Here are six pearls of wisdom, which you should always keep in mind when selecting colours:

1 Complete the skin tone test on page 99 and turn to pages 64–65 to find out which colours complement your skin tone.

2 Fifty shades of… Combine several tones of the same colour in one outfit.

3 Invest in colourful accessories: shoes, handbags, belts, scarves …

4 Look for colourful details on shirt cuffs, collars or socks to wear with your high heels.

5 Avoid wearing colours that are not part of your personal colour scheme close to your face.

6 Check the list of colour combinations and gain inspiration from some tried-and-tested pairings.

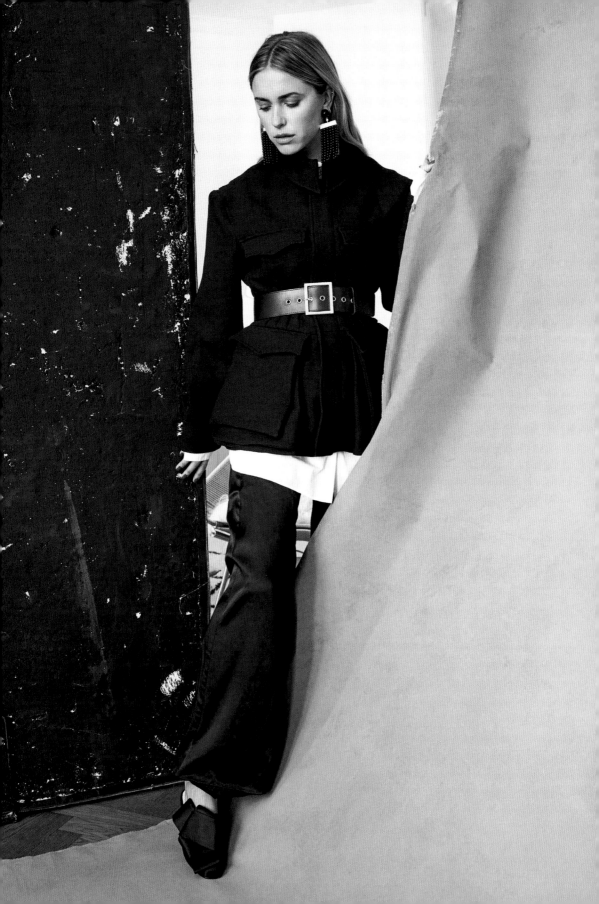

Knit,
Leather

& Layers

Due to the rather inhospitable Scandinavian climate, we have developed a preference for anything and everything that will keep us warm! Which is probably how we got to master the layer-on-layer concept without looking like the Michelin man. I will elaborate on the layer-on-layer concept a little later on, but firstly, let's talk about the Scandinavian ability to combine materials and textures in ways that brighten up even an all-black outfit.

Combining materials such as leather and knitwear creates contrasts and it allows one material to accentuate the other. For example, combine a leather biker jacket with something simple like a T-shirt and a pair of jeans. Then add a chunky knitted jumper, which, if only worn with T-shirt and jeans would give you a cosy and feminine look, and you will have created something interesting and unexpected. This may be fairly obvious to some people, but for others it may be something they've never considered before. Many of us buy our clothes as full outfits, and this may limit our ability to do something different, as we tend to get stuck with habits and become unable to see how to style a classic item in a new way. When you play around with new combinations you'll find you can use an expensive investment such as a leather jacket all year round.

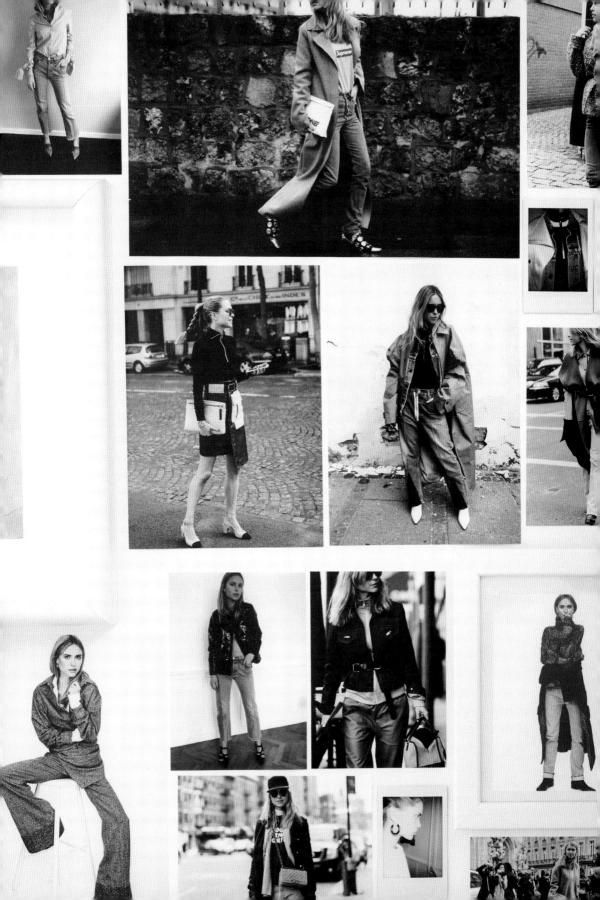

I love challenging my wardrobe– and indeed myself –
with new combinations, and I love it when I manage to
surprise myself. And yes, it still happens! This is also where I
reap the benefits of being a professional stylist and creative
consultant. Recently, I attended a show in New York by a brand
who are experts when it comes to creating new and exciting
variations of the classic shirt. The show included a shirt-on-
shirt combination with a lacquer polo neck underneath, which
immediately transformed it from a rather androgynous to a
really sexy look! Sometimes it's not about trailblazing new
materials or shapes; even obvious and simple combinations
can have the ability to surprise you. As this example shows,
wearing layer-on-layer means you can mix even more materials.

In Scandinavia, we grow up wearing several layers,
if only to stay warm in winter. My friend who was born and
raised in Los Angeles always says that she has no idea how we
manage to wear as many clothes as we do without looking like
giant balls of wool! It is indeed an art form. It's about knowing
your body and what suits you as it may otherwise go
horribly wrong.

Women are usually quite curvy, especially around the
stomach and hips, which is not always compatible with
layer-on-layer combinations of knitwear. Thank heavens for
heat-tech thermal under-tops from Uniqlo, which is the best
recommendation I can give for layering – to both women and
men. It's a bit like skiing underwear in that it retains body
heat, but it's not visible underneath a delicate knitted top.
It's a great starting point from which to embark on the layer-
on-layer technique in the cold winter months. These tops
come in various sleeve-lengths and they blend beautifully
with most outfits. You can even leave the cuffs sticking out
underneath a shirt with rolled-up sleeves or under a V-neck
knitted sweater.

Personally, I love polo necks. You can use them under dresses, woolly knitwear, shirts or tops – you name it! As long as they are a tight fit, they can seem almost slimming, for example, try a black polo neck under a white or colourful top. Then you can add yet another layer by wearing a blazer, which leaves the top of the polo neck sticking out. In this way, the jumper or knitted top is the colourful element while the blazer tones it all down a little, making for a more casual look.

Another great layer-on-layer idea for those cold winter evenings is wearing a simple polo neck or lace top with a round neck under a V-neck sweater, as this instantly adds femininity to the knitwear while also allowing you to use a summer top in winter.

Playing around with different layers continues to be a source of inspiration to me. Dresses worn over trousers is nothing new, although it's not a combination I'd ever wanted to try out myself – that is until Phoebe Philo of Céline showed us a really elegant version in her AW16 Collection. A sleeveless, knee-length satin-silk dress, draped at the sides, was worn over a sleeveless, thin, knitted polo neck and both were worn over a pair of wide woolly trousers. All items were the same utterly feminine and elegant cream colour. This inspired me to experiment with a silk-satin dress I would normally only ever wear in summer. Now, however, I use it more than ever. The combination of various materials and layers modernise your look, even if it is utterly simple.

I'm a huge fan of Phoebe Philo. Ever since 2008, the way she modernised vintage shapes has worked wonders for Céline. Before she started working there, Céline appeared a little dusty. However, Phoebe designs clothes based on her own wardrobe, which makes her collections stand out from the rest in a highly individual and minimalistic way. Her whole way of working is a perfect fit with the Scandinavian preference for streamlined aesthetics, and of course she then always adds a particular detail which makes it just that little bit more interesting.

Six Tips for the Layer-on-Layer Look

1 It's about striking a balance and creating harmony, so start off by looking at your body and defining your 'soft spots' – whether it's your hips, arms or waist.

2 Women with slim hips, broad shoulders or a voluptuous bosom should avoid large knitted jumpers. Instead, wear something tight-fitting such as the indispensable dark polo necks underneath a shirt or delicate silk top.

3 If your hips are wide or your legs heavy set, you can go wild with layer-on-layer of shirts and chunky knitwear underneath your leather jacket.

4 If you don't have much of a waist, a hip-length blazer over a delicate knitted top will make your torso appear longer than it is and thus remove focus from the midriff. A knee-length dress over a pair of wide trousers will also add volume below and thus beautifully curve your body.

5 Take 30 minutes to try out new combinations with what's already in your wardrobe, i.e. leather with knitwear or lace with wool. It takes a little time, but it'll save you money as you may discover some new looks without having to buy new clothes.

6 Break old habits and wear a summer dress in winter, either underneath a delicate knitted top or over a pair of trousers.

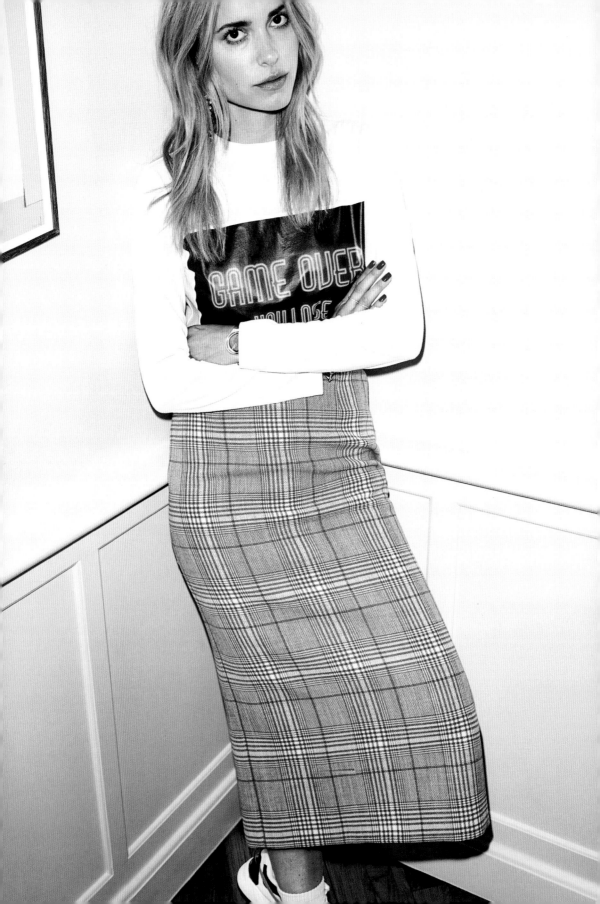

Keeping It Casual

To an outsider, the Scandinavian look may appear rather casual and minimalistic, but make no mistake, it's never accidental. Comfort ranks highly when we put together an outfit, but every little detail has been carefully considered, even when it looks as if we just quickly threw something on! The Scandinavian style equals confidence and tranquillity, which is what makes it so appealing.

We are great at combining various styles that either lift or tone-down an outfit, while also creating contrasts. One example is tracksuit bottoms, which you would normally only wear at home. I wore a pair during a fashion week in Paris with a casual printed T-shirt, a feminine leopard-print coat and a pair of sexy stilettos as the final touch. It may sound a little mad, but the various contrasts made this outfit work like a dream. I was comfortable and therefore totally confident. I could also have worn a sporty hoodie over a long dress, in order to turn the jogging outfit completely on its head. Another example would be an old, worn-out T-shirt worn with a classic pencil skirt and trainers. The T-shirt will neutralise the skirt's formal or matronly feel, and conversely the skirt upgrades the old T-shirt, making it suitable even for work.

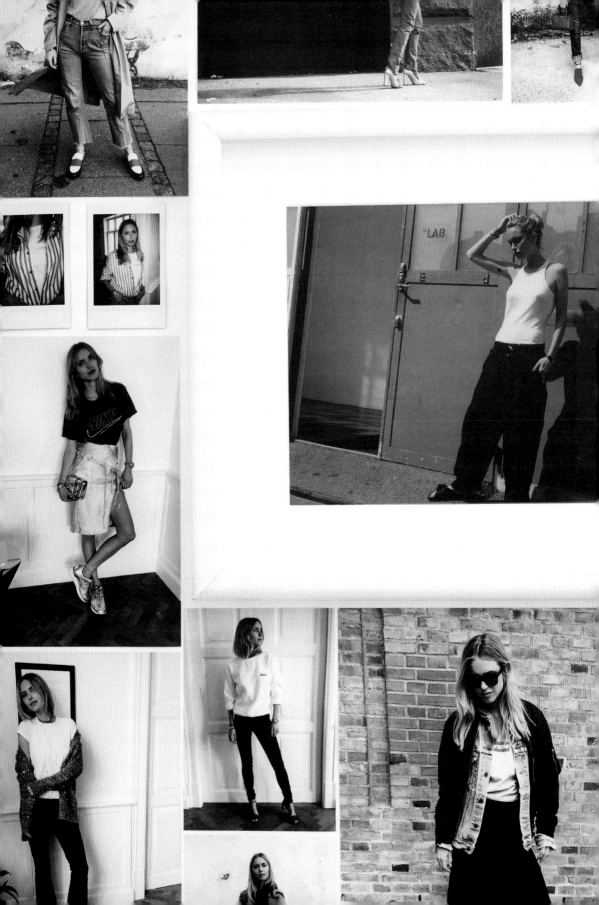

In this chapter, I'll look at items that most of us already have in our wardrobe, but which we might not have put together. Once you start thinking this way, it means you won't spend money on clothes you don't need, and you'll have more space in your wardrobe too! Once again, it's the philosophy of 'less is more'. I always have Coco Chanel's famous quotation at the back of my mind: 'Before you leave the house, look in the mirror and take one thing off'.

This is sound advice that I greatly appreciate, not least because we've all been there, wondering whether it's too early to flash the summer hat or whether you could have worn slightly less jewellery as you walk out the door. Basically, it's about feeling good without becoming overly casual – it's a delicate balance, which can be hard to maintain.

Here are some suggestions for combinations of classic items, which are either upgraded or toned down.

The Blazer

Wear it with a simple T-shirt or a hoodie to add a sporty contrast. If you're going for the more casual look, you can wear it over a chunky sweater. For the more feminine look, wear a knee-length dress underneath.

Trainers

Leave the high heels in the wardrobe and wear trainers with your classic outfit, which is then instantly toned down. You can also wear trainers with a delicate silk dress, which then becomes more sporty and suitable for everyday wear.

The White Shirt

Easily upgrade this item by adding a silk ribbon or tone it down by wearing it buttoned only half way over a thin top with a pair of jeans, i.e. use the shirt almost like a cardigan.

Suit Trousers

Roll the trouser legs up once or twice and wear coloured socks to create a great contrast to the classic look. You can easily upgrade the trousers by wearing them with a delicate lace camisole, which adds femininity to an otherwise masculine outfit.

As implied by the name, the pencil skirt is long and slender, fitted and it usually stops either just above or below the knee. It's a very classic shape, which enhances female curves. Wear it with an old T-shirt or a chunky knitted sweater to tone it down and reduce its feminine feel.

Pencil Skirt

Wear them on a weekday with a pair of old Levi's 501's or a pair of tracksuit bottoms and a simple top to create that perfect everyday look.

High Heels

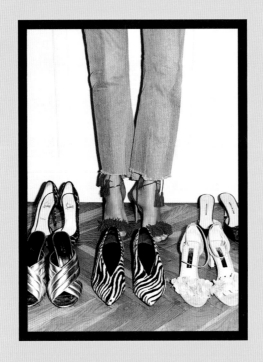

Chapter 8

My Precious

Accessories are the icing on the cake, and they can miraculously transform any look. Earlier, I mentioned the lack of colourful items in my wardrobe, except maybe for a knitted top or two. However, I made no mention of my shoes and handbags – they are definitely the noisiest items in there! I only have a few pairs of black shoes; all the others are colourful, metallic, peculiar or conspicuous. Is that a particularly Scandinavian thing? Well, yes and no – of course it depends on what you wear them with. If I wear a pair of red, fringed Aquazzura stilettos with a red handbag, it will be both eye-catching and feminine. If I wore some Gucci loafers or a pair of metallic trainers with a classic pencil skirt and a shirt it would make the look more interesting and also slightly androgynous.

When I get home from fashion weeks and look at street-style photos I'm always keeping an eye out for ideas of how to style my accessories in new and different ways. It's great to include an element of surprise in your look, and the best way to do this is with one of your accessories. I love shoes and handbags, (though I'm no competition for Carrie Bradshaw!) and they can be the safest bet, as they are easy to reuse and re-style.

With time, I've grown bolder when it comes to accessories, and not least when we're talking about shoes. I've discussed how important it is to have a solid, basic wardrobe, but that doesn't mean that I don't sometimes feel the urge to stand out from the crowd. That's when I put on a pair of Rupert Sanderson's iconic flower sandals on a grey Monday morning. Worn with a pair of old Levi's and a T-shirt, they are the definition of eye-catching!

Accessories can be an investment. At least that's what I happily tell myself each time I come home from Paris fashion week, and a pit stop at Céline or Chanel! It's very important to consider how you can upgrade your collection of accessories.

Firstly, check what you're missing in terms of shoes or handbags, and then consider what you need them for. Don't think that you can only wear your metallic, shiny high heels on New Year's Eve with an amazing ball gown. Use them with your everyday clothes, including a pair of old jeans and a sweatshirt. This will help you create exactly that comfy and confident look most people yearn for.

Regardless of price, you should always take good care of your possessions. Clothes and accessories require maintenance if you want them to last and hold their value, especially if one day you decide to sell them or hand them on to your daughter. I always carefully follow the washing instructions on the labels of my clothes; I know some of my favourites really won't benefit from a rough ride in the washing machine. Stains and smells can linger in clothes if you don't take action. So make sure you check your clothes before putting them back in the wardrobe. Pamper your woolly items by giving them a wool treatment once in a while, as this will help maintain the natural fat in wool, which makes it soft but also more durable.

The same goes for your leather shoes. Treat them with leather protection cream every once in a while, because leather is like skin, it needs 'lotion'. Rain, snow and salt will dry out leather. And your shoes will also look better when polished, as will your leather handbag. Remember to also resole your shoes not too long after you buy them. Soles on both cheap and expensive shoes are often not as durable as the ones you buy from the cobbler's.

Six Ways to Style Accessories

1
— Never decide to only use a fancy handbag on special occasions. Use it on weekdays as well as it will provide a lovely contrast to a comfy knitted sweater and a pair of casual trainers.

2
— Make sure you feel comfortable and able to dance all night in every single pair of heels in your wardrobe. Once you find the high heels that work for you; stick with them. This will also help you avoid the numerous mistakes that only end up covered in dust in the bottom of your wardrobe. Finding out which heels will work for you is easy – all you have to do is check to see whether your instep aligns with the sole of the shoe. If there's space between your instep and the sole, the heels are too high for you.

3
— Challenge yourself and buy a pair of red or blue stilettos. They are a perfect match for the Scandinavian colour scheme, and they equal instant attention.

4
— Over the last few seasons, the classic loafer has developed into a hybrid between a loafer and a slipper, thanks to Alessandro Michele for Gucci. I love this subtle change, because it equals a fresh take on a classic shoe, which suits Scandinavian fashion perfectly. Go for the backless version or a classic pair; only don't buy black or brown, but choose grey, blue, red or white ones. You can get loafers in practically every price range, from high-street prices and upwards.

5
— The belt is a dear and useful friend. Don't limit them to jeans and trousers – belts can also add a highly feminine touch to our layer-on-layer outfits. Thin or wide, either will do, but the final look will differ markedly. Try using a thin belt with your coat, cardigan or over a delicate dress. You could also opt for a plaited piece of string or a ribbon, if you want a slightly more dressed-up look. If you want a more feminine shape and an explicit waistline, wear a wide belt. You could pair it with a chunky knitted jumper, an oversized man's shirt or as a smooth transition from top to skirt.

6
— Red lipstick is a classic, and has helped lift my look on many occasions when I'm a little run down, especially during my numerous fashion week marathons where sleep is never at the top of my list. The red colour complements the colder nuances in Scandinavian fashion, and in a split second you get a feminine and sexy upgrading of our otherwise androgynous look.

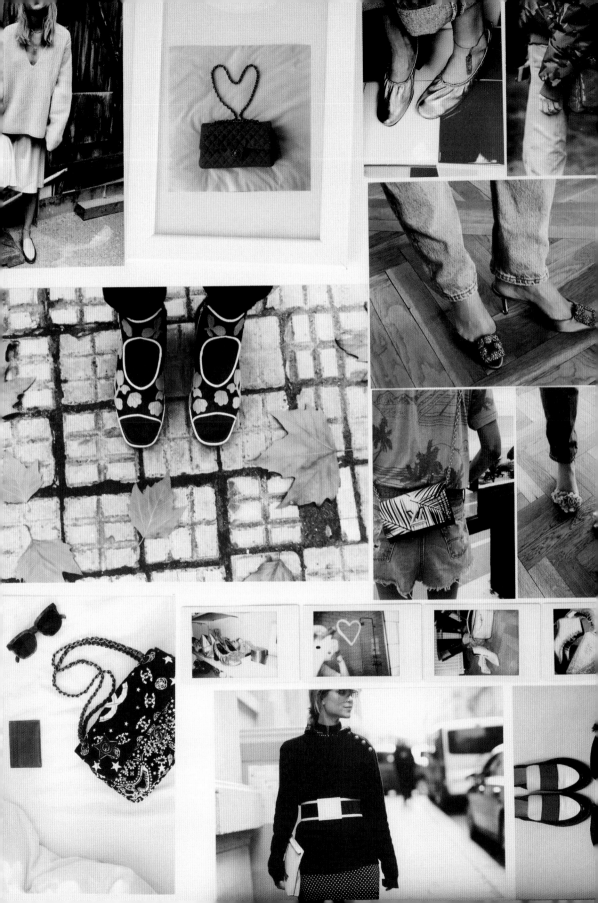

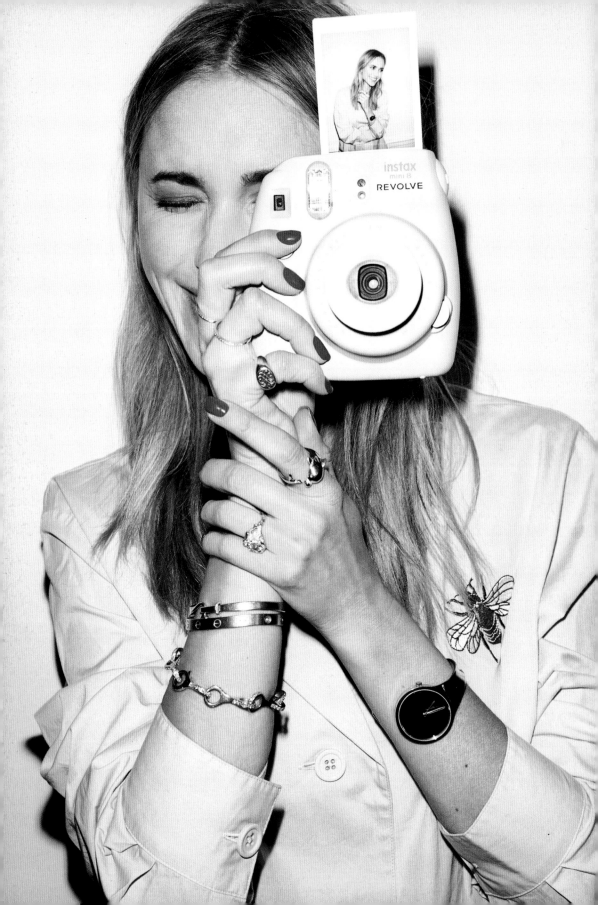

Bling Hotline

Something we do particularly well in Scandinavia is jewellery; thanks to our talented jewellers more than anything. They have really led the way when it comes to creating inspiring jewellery that most people can afford.

Jewellery effortlessly and quite elegantly adds personality to any look. It's an eye-catching detail that will upgrade any outfit. The latest trend where rings are worn on every finger joint, ears are lined with cuffs, and delicate chains are stacked up around our necks just goes to show how easy it is to customise your style by mixing and matching jewellery. Traditionally, jewellery was kept for 'best' and was only worn on special occasions; now we wear it 365 days a year. Jewellery becomes an integral part of you, and this makes you unique.

I'm delighted to see these new tendencies spreading worldwide, as jewellery is one of the many details I feel passionately about, and it is also very much part of my brand. I actually feel quite naked if I'm not wearing my jewellery. That's not to say that I walk around looking like a Christmas tree, but I do like experimenting with jewellery, particularly combining different styles in a conspicuous way.

When I had my 'turning 30' crisis and decided that I should get my nose pierced and add four more piercings to my ears, it's safe to say that I went a little overboard! The nose ring went after only a month, but I've used my ear piercings ever since. I love to wear a row of pearls or a collection of hoops in my ears, as they add a little edge to my otherwise rather classic look. I also go through periods when I wear the same jewellery day after day – even in the evening. The jewellery becomes almost an extension of me and my look. As time goes by, I seem to wear different jewellery less and less. Some of my jewellery has sentimental value; like my engagement ring, for instance, which my partner designed in collaboration with one of my favourite Danish designers. Though I do like to add contrast in the shape of a more minimalist ring or bracelet. This makes my overall look a little more fun and playful.

Experimenting with jewellery, and discovering favourite pieces, is a lifelong adventure. If you don't know how to start, here are a few tips:

Gold or Silver?
(Or Both?)

Personally, I'm very fond of gold, as gold goes really well with my skin tone and style. It took me a number of years to discover this – and naturally, I also had to save up to be able to afford to buy gold jewellery as it is, after all, a little more expensive than silver. The general rule is that gold suits warmer skin tones while silver complements a colder skin tone. If you don't know whether your skin tone is warm or cold, check out the tips below:

If your skin looks golden, beige or yellowish, your skin tone is warm. If your skin tone is more pink or rose, then your skin tone is cold.

If you have olive or chocolate coloured eyes, your skin tone is warm; if your eyes are icy blue or greyish, your skin tone is cold.

You can simply hold a piece of gold or silver jewellery up against your face to check which piece livens up your face more. If it's gold, your skin tone is warm, if it's silver, your skin tone is cold.

You can also test your skin tone by holding something that's off-white up against your face followed by something completely white. If the off-white tone is better for you, your skin tone is warm, if on the other hand, white suits you better then your skin tone is cold.

These are just guidelines to help you get started.

What's most important is feeling comfortable with what you're wearing. And do you even have to wear either gold OR silver? Of course not, you can easily mix different types of metal, which will provide you with a more playful look, as contrasts highlight each other.

Creating a solid collection of jewellery takes time.

So always choose carefully and save up, because investing in silver and gold is never a bad idea. Their value is more or less constant and they'll last for ever. Another tip is to keep an eye on what's on sale at auctions, where you can often find a beautiful piece of vintage jewellery in search of a new owner.

I'm very fond of designers such as Orit Elhanati. She combines her Israeli background and Scandinavian simplicity in a highly original way. The results are quite unique and wonderfully organic. Sophie Bille Brahe is another one of my favourite designers who masters the delicate balance between simple and classic, while still being modern and cool. And we must not forget Georg Jensen, where they have developed their collections considerably over the last few years, moving away from heavy silver jewellery, producing some truly elegant and modern designs. I wear my Georg Jensen jewellery every day; I never take it off. Trine Tuxen also makes beautiful gold and silver medallions, delicate loop rings and lovely ear bullets.

One accessory that I've stubbornly used for as long as I can remember my wristwatch. I started wearing a Pink Panther watch when I turned eight, and over the years, I've slowly upgraded to slightly more refined designs, which I have saved up for or been given as birthday presents. However, buying a watch doesn't have to be a huge investment. Skagen Watches have some really nice ones; classic, timeless watches made of steel and leather.

To me, watches belong in the 'bling-bling' category.

It used to be mainly men who concerned themselves with watches, but over time, women have become more and more interested. Watches have actually become a collector's item for me, and I've become rather nerdy in my attitude towards them! In fact, I'll even admit to believing that your choice of watch defines you and your style. Personally, I love the more masculine watches as they create a great contrast to my many, very feminine pieces of jewellery.

Details and jewellery are important to the Scandinavian look, as this is one place where our obsession with design and form can manifest itself. Keep this in mind when you want to bling-up your basic wardrobe!

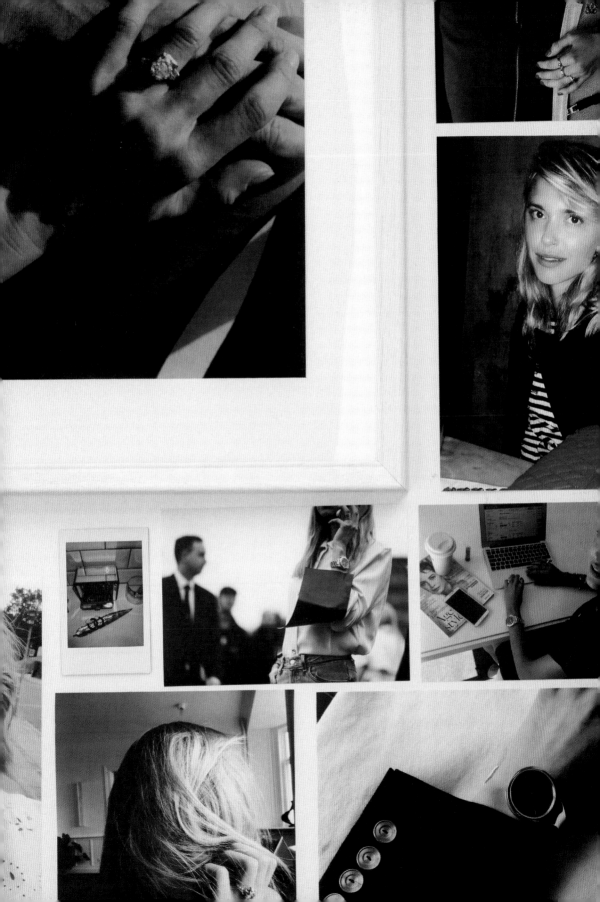

Do's

& Don'ts

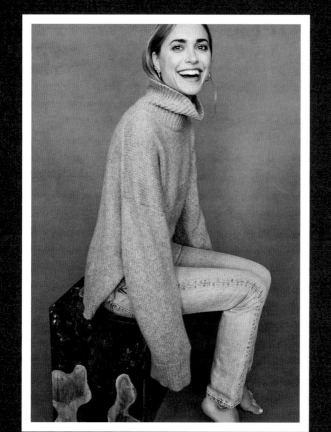

Do's

There are many ways of styling essential items in a Scandinavian wardrobe, so it might feel a little overwhelming when you first start to experiment with a Scandi approach to style, and finding your own look. I've tried to make it easier by putting together a list of Do's and Don'ts:

1 Remember, less is more – a simple outfit does not equal a boring outfit.

2 Always choose quality over quantity – but also keep in mind that quality does not merely equal expensive designer brands.

3 It's all in the details – always look for unusual new details and integrate them in a way you like.

4 Use more jewellery – it adds personality.

5 Build a solid basic wardrobe – this will help you avoid clothes' crises.

6 Use colours that suit your skin tone.

7 Mix materials – it creates contrasts and freshens your look.

8 Layer-on-layer adds more dimensions to your outfit.

9 Choose comfort over everything else.

10 Use eye-catching accessories.

Don'ts

I actually don't comply with some of fashion's absolute don'ts, which is also why I won't give you any. Fashion is a constantly evolving and innovative industry. Old trends I had long since sworn I'd never wear have become personal favourites. This usually happens when the right designer leaves their mark on a well-known item, or simply as a result of getting older and our personal tastes evolving. My mother's black lacquer jacket with shoulder pads from the 1980s always used to be an embarrassment to me, but today, I wish she'd kept it, so I could have inherited it! Another example is the aforementioned Mom jeans (see page 47), which I never thought I'd come to appreciate, as they give you the longest bottom ever. Neither would I have ever thought that socks in a pair of Jesus sandals, à la Marni Fussbett, would be something I'd want to wear, but I have to admit that it's an utterly comfortable trend, which I have embraced.

Even the dreaded H20 sandal is back, only now Stine Goya has added a chic gold rim, and Ganni have created a Buffalo boot, which in many ways is as ugly as I remember, yet they have managed to make it cool and street again.

So, never say die! Although I won't give you any don'ts, there are some things that I do try to avoid:

1 Thigh-high boots with miniskirts or mini-dresses. This simply doesn't work for me. Conversely, thigh-high boots go really well with a pair of jeans or knee-length dresses and skirts.

2 Corset tops aren't really my favourites. You can wear them over a shirt or T-shirt, but never on their own.

3 Poor quality basic items made of purely artificial materials are best avoided. This sort of fabric doesn't 'breathe', and basically, they're just not very comfortable.

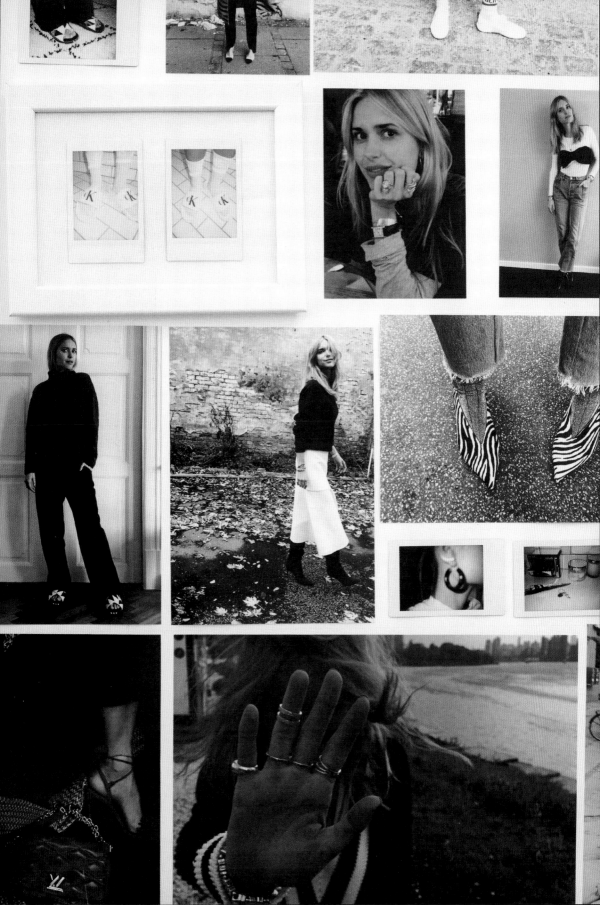

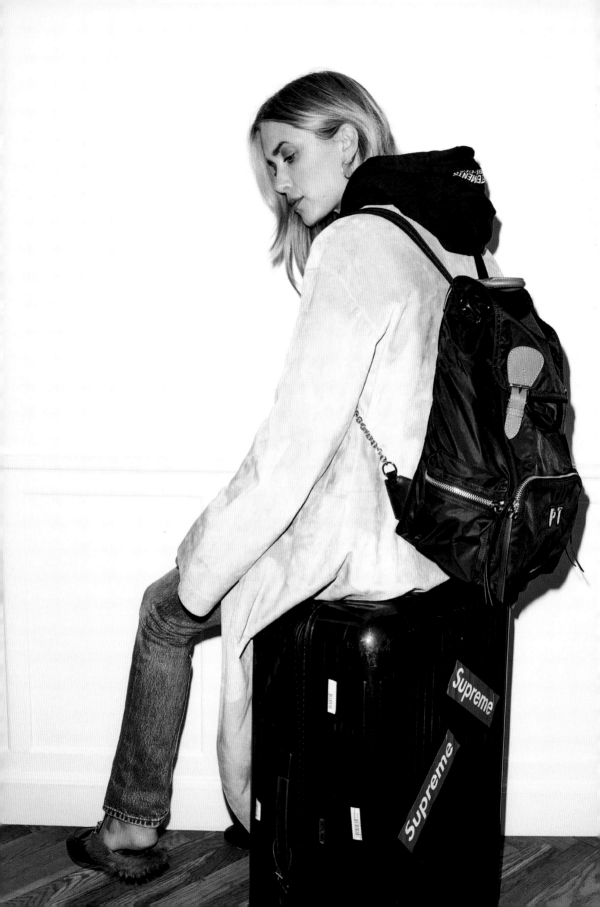

Go

On the

Go

Had you asked me two years ago, I would never have predicted that I'd be travelling as much as I do, but that's one of the by-products of living in Denmark. Fortunately, I love travelling, whether I'm going to a fashion week somewhere or just working in another country. And on some level, my many journeys have made the world feel a little smaller.

When I arrive somewhere new, I always try to walk around rather than take a taxi, Uber or train. Walking helps me find my bearings in a new city and I get inspiration from watching people on the streets. I always come across new shops, cafés or galleries that I would never have noticed had I not walked past them. Exploring calms me down, and it fuels my confidence, even when I'm merely walking from one show location to the next. It also gives me time to think about the various projects in my head, as being creative takes time and space – you cannot create on command.

In order to widen my horizons, I always include at least one cultural event in my travels. It can be anything from a local exhibition to a theatre performance, which always boosts my imagination and creates a greater understanding of – and insight into – other cultures.

Furthermore, I often meet new and exciting people – new acquaintances who sometimes become wonderful friends. Some of the people I have met on my travels have proved great sources of inspiration, which I'm eternally grateful for.

You'd think that, by now, I'd be able to compete in one of those 'how-to-pack-your-suitcase' competitions, seeing as I'm constantly on the move! Have you seen Louis Vuitton's amazing packing guide: 'The Art of Packing', where they manage to pack an entire wardrobe into a tiny bag? I am nowhere near that!

However, I am good at preparing what to bring, even if it sometimes (okay, always) results in my suitcase being overweight.

When I prepare for my annual fashion week marathon, nothing makes its way into my suitcase by accident. I plan every outfit beforehand, so I don't waste space on items I won't wear. Though I do often pack more outfits than I need, so I can change my mind along the way. Planning outfits in advance gives me a better overview of all the items I'm taking and it definitely saves time once you get to your destination, whether it's a business or leisure trip.

The main thing to remember is that it's all about being able to reuse as many items as possible by combining them in different ways. And this is when your basic wardrobe comes in really handy, because, as we've seen, a great basic wardrobe allows you to change your entire look by simply twisting tiny details. Perfect for when you are away from home.

In other words, preparation is halfway to being packed. Which naturally also means that you should allocate more time to preparing than you are probably used to! In the past when I went away, I would end up with five pairs of jeans, 10 pairs of shoes and only two tops in my holiday suitcase. It was always utterly chaotic. But then I grabbed the bull by the horns and changed my ways.

A good tip is to take photos of your different outfits, as this will enable you to remember what you were thinking at home. You can then pack each item individually, which takes up less space than trying to pack a whole outfit together.

Finally, always take underwear, a top and a pair of high heels in your hand luggage, just in case your suitcase is delayed by a day or two.

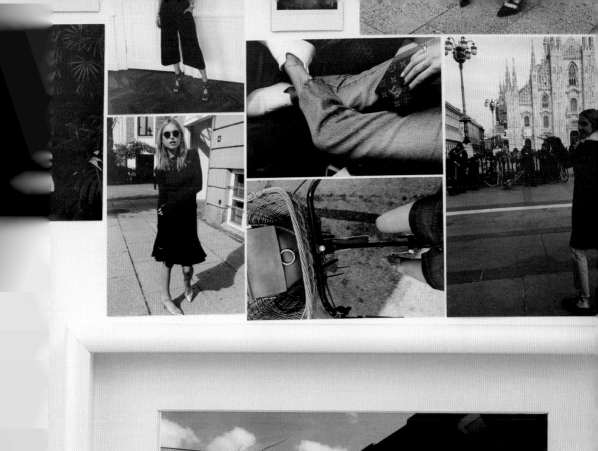
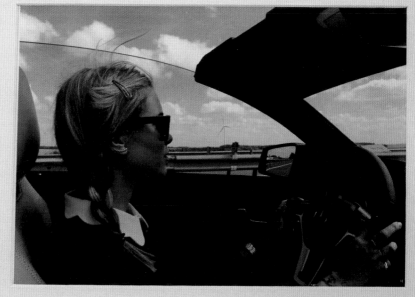
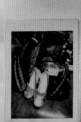
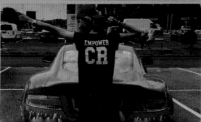
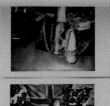
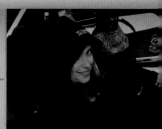

Chapter 12

My Inspiration

When I wake up in the morning and don't know what to wear, when I lack inspiration for a fashion series or even my own home, Leandra Medine and Vanessa Traina are the first people I'll check out on Instagram and online, because they ooze personality and sometimes they even add that tiny twist of Scandinavian aesthetics.

I've followed both women for years, and I'm eternally grateful for everything they have taught me. Today, I know them both personally, and we share stories as well as tips and tricks for our wardrobe.

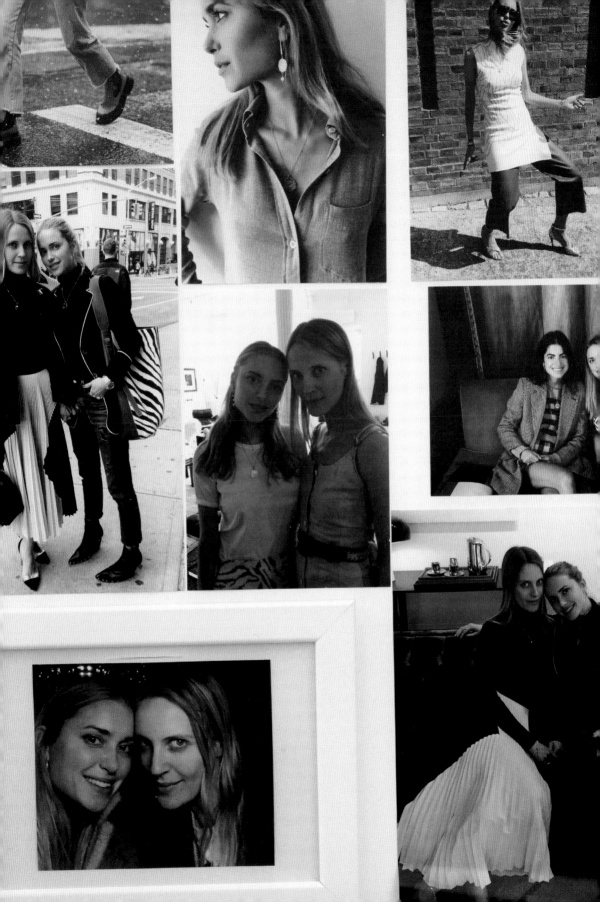

Leandra Medine

You may know Leandra better by the name of her successful blog, Manrepeller, where she writes about trends and beauty in a highly unusual, inspiring and humorous way, sometimes adding entertaining quizzes and stories from her personal life. She is also the author of the book *Seeking Love, Finding Overalls*, published in 2013.

I've followed Leandra ever since she started Manrepeller, and I've always been fascinated by her unique, inspiring and surprising clothes combinations. She lives in New York, but we always meet and catch up during fashion weeks.

We met in my favourite hotel in New York, my home away from home, the Soho Grand:

Pernille: Can you describe the Scandinavian style in just a few words?

Leandra: Minimalist, yet interesting; surprising, simple and tailored.

P: I agree! What in your opinion constitutes the essence of Scandinavian style?

L: I believe that the reason I'm attracted to the Scandinavian style is because it's not 'crazy', it's extremely inspiring and always surprising, usually because of one single detail that renders the entire look unique. It's not merely the 'sweater and trousers' combination, it's a sweater with rolled-up sleeves, revealing a row of beautiful bracelets, topped with that blonde hair. It's a different approach to thinking about fashion.

P: Yes, the details definitely decide the final outfit. But what are the key items in your mind, when we talk about Scandinavian style?

L: Trainers! When I started wearing trainers in New York, three years ago, I felt very Scandinavian. Perhaps because so many of the Scandinavian tourists always wear trainers when they visit, and I thought that they looked so tall and cool in their Chanel trainers, like the Danish model, Caroline Brasch Nielsen.

P: I didn't see that answer coming. I always thought that we embraced the trainer thanks to you guys. But then again, you're right in pointing out that girls like Caroline Brasch Nielsen really master the trainer look. And we are possibly more practical minded in Scandinavia, because we love comfort. How do you integrate Scandinavian style into your own wardrobe?

L: I follow you on Instagram!

P: Ha! You're making me blush, what a compliment! But apart from my Instagram?

L: It's difficult to say, but you'll frequently see me in trainers now. And sometimes, I wish that my hair was blonde like you Scandinavian girls. Then I could wear darker clothes. With my hair colour, I feel it might get a little too dark-on-dark. When I feel a little dressed up, I ask myself; 'what would I wear to make people think I was Scandinavian?' Then I'd probably remove some of the items, the stuff that would make it seem a little OTT, and exchange it for something slightly more classic. What I like about well-dressed Scandinavian women is their ability to make a black sweater and jeans look interesting. No one else can do that. And I really like denim.

P: Me too, I'm a huge fan of denim! Possibly even a little addicted… Well, I've prepared a quick quiz for you. I'll say a word, and answer with whatever pops into your head. Here goes: minimalism?

L: Can be good. If you're a slightly boring person, it's not great. It's about personality, really. If you're a vibrant and colourful type who dresses minimalistically, it can be incredibly elegant, because of the groovy contrast.

P: Yeah, we're both very fond of contrasts! Next word: stripes?

L: You can never go wrong with stripes. It's an easy way to make a fancy outfit more casual, and it provides an exciting contrast, which I really like to incorporate in my looks. Looking fancy in a casual way is what Scandinavian women do so well. If I'm going to a wedding, I'm not the type of person who would wear a matching top and skirt, as it would feel way too 'matching' and 'suity'. I would immediately exchange the top for a go-to striped shirt to create a contrast.

P: I'll keep that in mind! Next word: Vikings?

L: Cool hats, I want one!

P: Danish pastry?

L: Don't get me started; I love Danish pastry, covered in sugar and nuts.

P: I actually knew that, only you hide it well. Next word: layer-on-layer?

L: Well, that's totally my motto; more is more. I love wearing layers.

P: Bicycle?

L: A good excuse to wear spandex?

P: Navy blue?

L: Makes me think of Phoebe Philo for Céline. I love navy and black together, only when I was young, my mother would say that those two colours didn't match, so I was in denial for five years.

P: Lastly, would you share a tip that you yourself use right now?

L: Currently, I'm thinking ballerina shoes with baggy trousers. And I'm thinking socks in shoes and slip dresses with lace-up sandals.

Vanessa Traina

I've been Vanessa Traina's biggest fan for years. I LOVE her style, aesthetics and taste. Vanessa grew up in San Francisco and she's the daughter of the author Danielle Steel. She used to model and then embarked on a career as a stylist, and now she's a creative consultant for Alexander Wang and Joseph Altuzarra, among others. In 2013, she launched a web shop, The Line, as well as a showroom in New York, which is designed like an apartment, where you'll find everything your heart desires in terms of art, furniture and clothes.

Vanessa and I came to know one another because I sent her an invitation for a Georg Jensen event I was hosting in New York via Instagram. She answered straightaway to say that unfortunately, she wasn't able to make it, but should we meet for coffee instead? We instantly became friends and now we meet up all the time, be it at fashion weeks or private get-togethers. Vanessa is always first on my list when I'm in New York.

Pernille: Can you describe the Scandinavian style in just a few words?

Vanessa: Streamlined, elegant and functional! And then there's your light colouring. I could definitely pass as Scandinavian; I'm blonde with blue eyes.

P: What do you consider essentially Scandinavian?

V: To me it's about fit and material. I wouldn't necessarily call it minimalistic, but more of a great basic wardrobe. It's all about the cut and construction, which makes it all come together.

P: How do you integrate the Scandinavian style into your own wardrobe?

V: I think of all the fundamental styles in a wardrobe. Some call them basic, but that's not how I see it. They are incredibly important, exactly because they are the items upon which you build everything else. It's a bit like the foundation in your make-up.

P: So what are the key items that spring to mind when we talk about Scandinavian style?

V: Obviously my 'basic' wardrobe, which consists of the best items in any category, such as a cashmere sweater, quality jeans, fitted blazer and a streamlined coat. I'm also constantly drawn to pure lines and shapes, which are the incarnation of Scandinavian style.

P: I've prepared a quick quiz for you. I'll say a word, and you'll tell me what pops into your head. Here goes: sailor stripes?

V: I'm thinking Breton stripes.

P: Of course you're thinking of French stripes, but we're very good with stripes too. Perhaps with a slightly more maritime approach. Danish pastry?

V: Well, that makes me think of calories – Danish pastry is most certainly a guilty pleasure!

P: Layer-on-layer?

V: Practical, functional and necessary.

P: Cycling?

V: Makes me think of Amsterdam!

P: Well that's because you haven't been to Denmark yet, because it's the preferred method of transportation for most city-dwellers there too. How about Vikings?

V: The hat, without a shadow of doubt.

P: That's what Leandra said – I'll have to get you guys one! What's your best styling tip?

V: My best tip is having a great tailor. A tailored fit will lift even the most casual style.

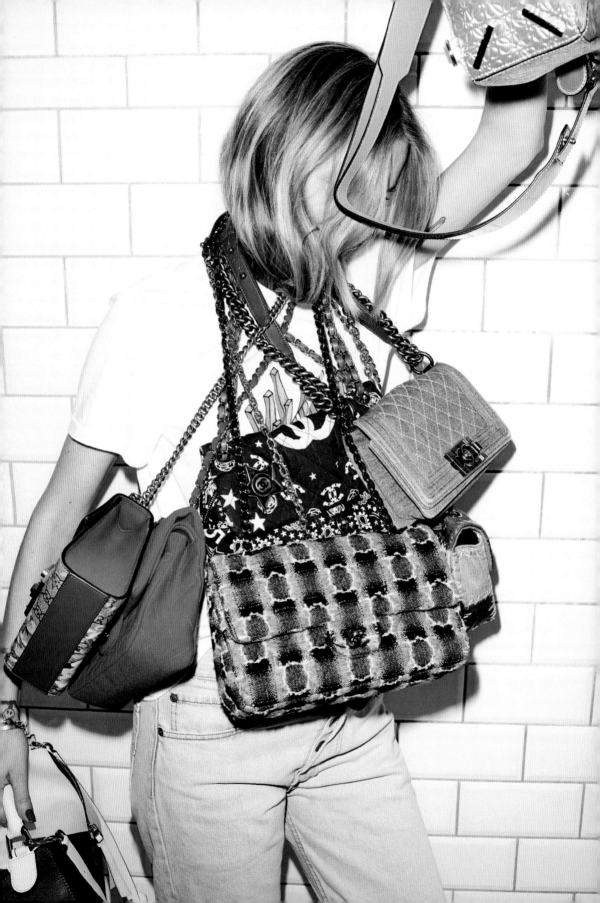

Where Did All My Go?

Money

(I know I made some)

Some people invest in stocks and shares and others in cars. Throughout the years, I've invested a lot of money in my wardrobe, including handbags and iconic items, which I will most likely keep for ever, because they are of sentimental value to me. I have everything from an iconic Chanel handbag to a timeless Céline coat. Each item seemed to somehow mysteriously end up in my suitcase when I was on my many travels! Paris is especially bad for my bank balance, as I usually end fashion week by treating myself to something nice.

Now, you may think that I spend all my time shopping, but I carefully plan each investment – and I save up for them – totally old school!

I asked my lovely friend Hannah Løffler what she thinks sums up my approach to investing in my wardrobe. She said this:

'Twice a year, you know that Ms Methodical is getting excited about the coming "flea market season". She eagerly stuffs her bags with everything she believes should no longer reside in her wardrobe. Pernille loves presenting her stuff; stacking things and hanging them neatly on racks, and then she watches people as they swarm in. She knows that the more old stuff she manages to sell, the more new stuff she can afford next time she's in Paris. Pernille is very disciplined, and she'll put every penny she makes at the flea market aside and then patiently await another visit to Céline or Chanel.'

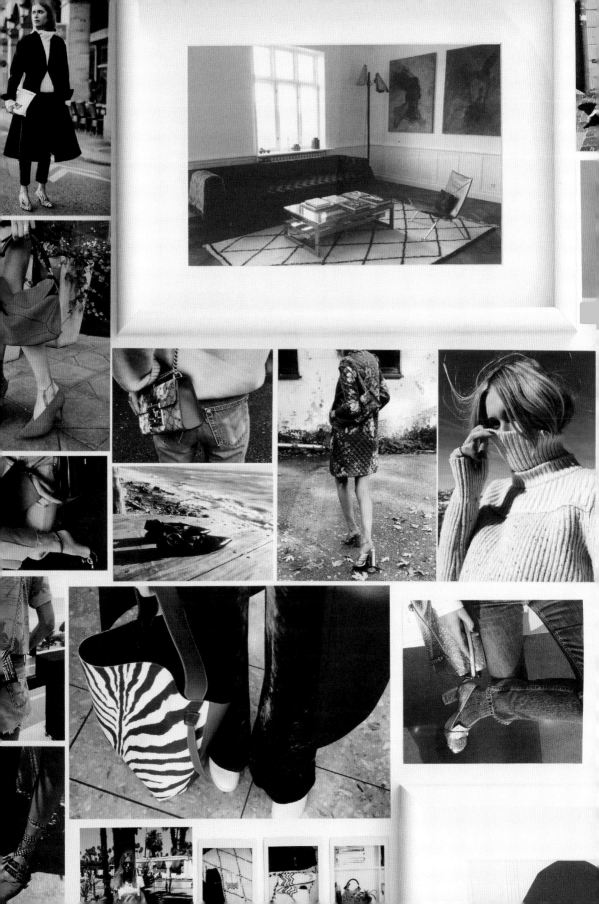

Like everybody else, of course I sometimes manage to overspend, and I blame online shopping. All sorts of temptations end up in my inbox on a daily basis. I don't fall prey to temptation that often really, but once I start browsing through webpages, I also start looking for clothes from the previous season, and then I start regretting that I didn't get them first time around… That's the lure of online shopping; you can get whatever your heart desires!

During the last couple of years, I've also made some seriously great second-hand finds. However, I'll also be the first to admit that it's rarely (never) in a shop, but rather on websites such as Vestiaire Collective, The Real Deal Collection or Resee. There you'll find anything from classic Burberry trench coats to runway samples from Nicolas Ghesquière, when he worked for Balenciaga. These are top-of-the-range luxury items, but online you just might be able to find them at reasonable prices.

I've also made a number of great investments during the sales, although it's important to keep a clear head in these situations, or you may be tempted to buy all sorts of things that you don't actually need and that you can't really afford either. There are many times that I've come home with something and then thought: 'Oh God, I'm never going to wear that horror!' Then I get quite upset with myself, because I haven't saved any money at all, instead I've spent it on rubbish.

However, I've also learnt a lot from my mistakes, and now I tend to approach sales shopping from a more sensible angle. First of all, I'll have a serious think about what I actually need and only then will I go shopping. Sales are a great time to look for items for your basic wardrobe. For example, I've bought several blazers, shirts and knitwear in the sales, which I today consider some of my best buys. If I have time, I'll visit the shops I like to browse before the sales begin. Then when the sales start, I can go straight for the items I want and not waste time fighting for inconsequential things I don't want anyway!

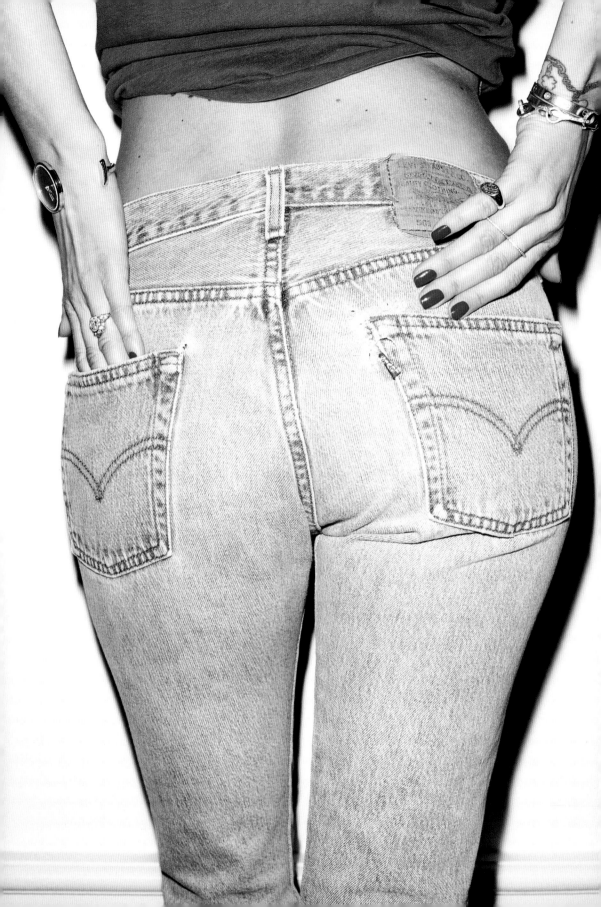

My Top 10 Best Buys

My absolute best buys throughout the years include everything from sales scoops to high-street items. These are the absolute staples of my wardrobe, and hopefully they will inspire you to think about what you already have, and what might be a great addition to your own style.

1 A camel or beige coloured cashmere knitted turtleneck jumper from Céline with long sleeves and a boxy-fit. It's a timeless classic, which I'll continue to wear until it falls apart because it goes with everything, from a pair of cut-off denim shorts in summer to a woolly pencil skirt in winter.

2 Vintage Levi's jeans that cost me DKK 100 (around £11) on eBay. They are coming apart at the seams, they've been worn so much. They've also been mentioned multiple times in this book, which shows you just how important they are to me!

3 White Reebok trainers; a perfect combination of classic tennis shoe and a retro 1990s look.

4 Miu Miu mules with bows. At first I regretted buying them, but then I discovered that they have that eye-catching factor, which immediately gives your everyday look a personal twist.

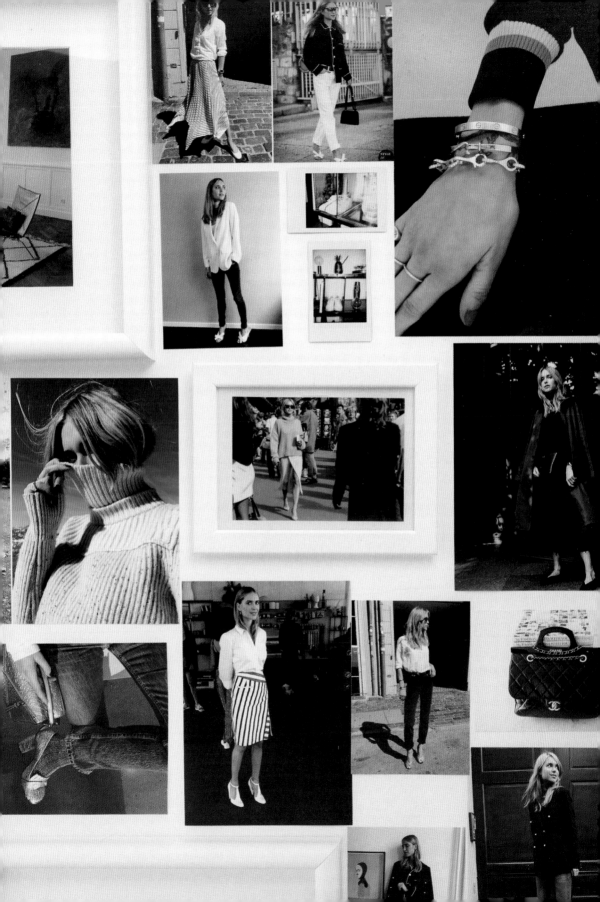

5 A Chanel handbag. It's very ladylike and classic, but size matters and that's why it's my favourite handbag. I was helping a friend buy a handbag when I saw it, and so I hadn't calculated on impulse buying anything in that price range. I tried really hard to convince myself that I didn't need it, but I struck a deal with myself: if I could fit my laptop into it, it would be a perfect handbag for work. So a few hours later, I returned to the shop, laptop in hand, and naturally, it fitted like a glove. I was left with no choice, I 'had' to buy it.

6 A Céline blazer with white pearl buttons. It's possibly one of the best sales purchases I've ever made. I saw it in a shop called Storm, the day before the sales started.

7 A gold chain with diamonds from Georg Jensen. I've worn it ever since I spotted it during a shoot. I simply had to own it. It's a perfect combination of classic chain with a touch of bling-bling.

8 A white shirt from Nué Notes with a Mandarin collar. I never have to iron it and that's why it's always in my suitcase when I'm travelling. The delicate material gives it a feminine look and sometimes I wear a lace bra in a contrasting colour underneath, which makes for a perfect transition to eveningwear.

9 A navy blue coat from Comme des Garçons, called the Luna tent on account of its A- shape. It was yet another sales find, and I actually bought it as a practical coat that I would only use for trips to our summerhouse or on Sunday walks around the lakes of Copenhagen. However, it has become a coat I wear more often than almost any other coat, not least because it's incredibly comfortable and it's also a little different without sticking out too much.

10 A striped pencil skirt from Altuzarra, which is my go-to skirt when I find myself in a clothes' crisis. Its classic shape makes it timeless, yet it's incredibly feminine and sexy, not least because of its high slit.

The Death
of the ~~Dress~~ Code

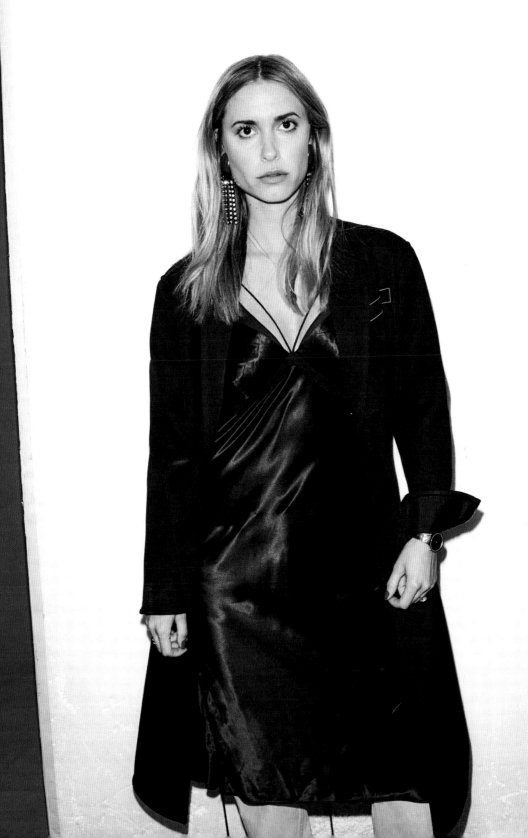

Traditional ideas about how we should dress during the day, in the evening, at work or on special occasions have changed over the last few years. Old jeans or trainers are just as common now as eveningwear as cocktail dresses and expensive high heels are popular as everyday shoes. Anything goes – and that's incredibly liberating!

And why should it have to be so predictable in the first place?

Ten years ago, you wouldn't see hoodies or trainers on the catwalk, but fortunately, these days traditional fashion houses are much more open to a modern mix. Which is also why, on the flip-side, we no longer leave our fancier items – such as dresses, party tops and stilettos – gathering dust at home. It's all about balancing our desire to stand out, while simultaneously fitting in; feeling comfortable and being dressed appropriately for the occasion.

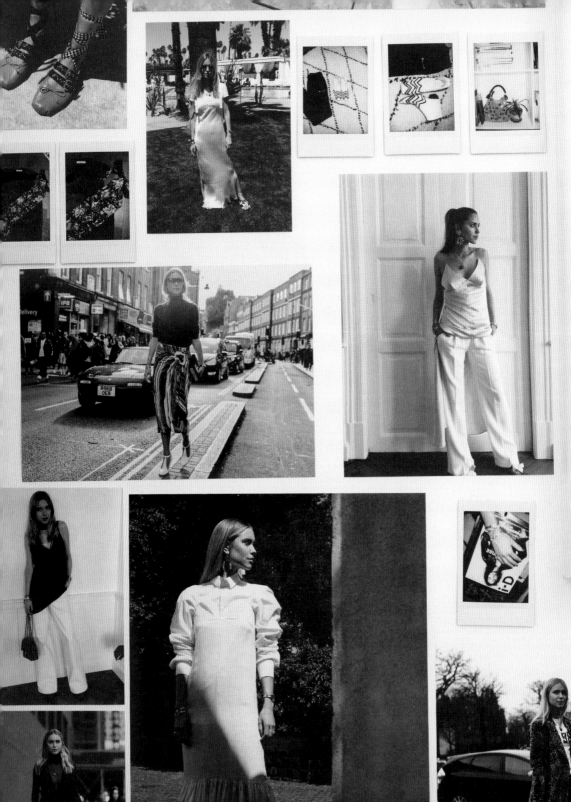
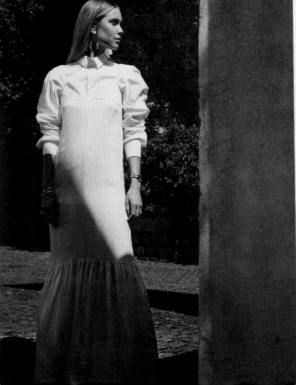
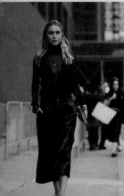
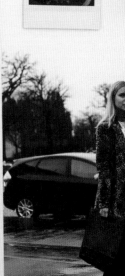

Work Wear

I would save both time and money if I had some sort of defined work uniform such as a suit or a white lab coat! Recently, I had a rather amusing conversation with my agent, Hannah, about work wear. We had a meeting with a future client, and to my horror, I watched Hannah walking towards me dressed in old, worn-out trainers, a washed-out hunting jacket, which she's had since she was 16 years old, and maternity trousers that should never have been let out of the house! It had comfort written all over, and it was just a tad too relaxed for my taste. However, she was beaming, because she felt really good, and that shifted everyone's focus from what she was wearing. Work wear is truly a question of balancing your mood on any given day, whether it's wearing a short miniskirt because you feel on top of the world on a Monday, or whether a more low-key T-shirt and jeans are called for.

I often wear high heels when I have an important meeting, because heels feed my self-confidence and sense of power.

Social Occasions

Lots of us will have received an invitation to an event where the small print includes a dress code, like 'cocktail dresses' or 'black tie'. To me, it's a great relief, because then you don't have to worry about whether you're over or under dressed. I hate it when there's no indication of what to wear, because it leaves guests undecided and often results in a safe bet: jeans, a nice shirt and high heels.

So, am I saying that we should always wear what we feel like? Wearing something you like has a tremendous effect on your radiance and confidence. However, I still think it's important to push the boundaries and step out of one's comfort zone – so long as you don't try to completely change your style or spend a fortune. This can include anything from colourful shoes to bling-bling earrings from any high-street shop. Start looking around and get inspired!

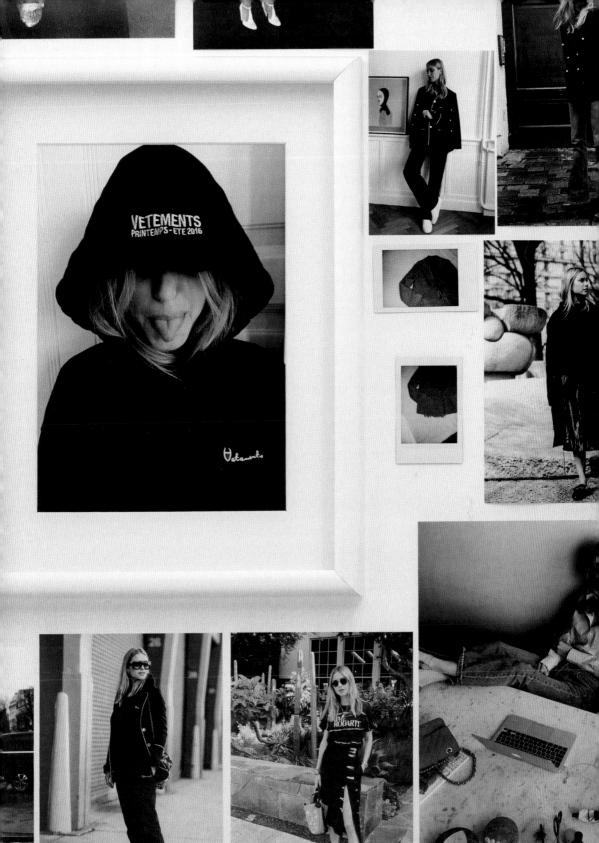

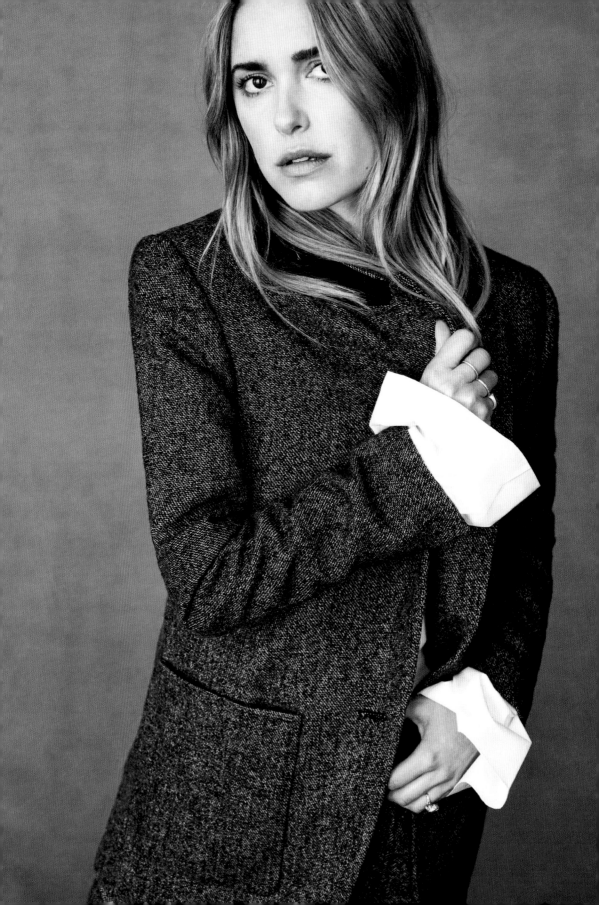

It's

Mix

All

in

the

I've always been a firm believer in high-street brands, because quality does not have to equal expensive. Over the last few years, many of the high-street brands that I love have greatly improved the quality of their items. A few years back, I did a shoot for a British high-street chain, REISS, a brand I wasn't particularly familiar with at the time. It was a series inspired by men's fashion, and – because I am pretty partial to the androgynous look – I ended up mixing the women and men's collections, which turned out to be a lot of fun. Afterwards, I bought a man's cashmere polo neck in the smallest size available, and it's been my favourite knitwear ever since. It's extremely good quality; it does not lose its shape and there's no fluff. You can make some amazing finds in the men's department in high-street shops.

In my opinion, mixing cheap and expensive items will give you a more personalised look. I don't find it terribly inspiring when people buy the entire catwalk outfit or a formulated outfit from ZARA. Instead, mix in some of your grand old classics, your best purchases, or some great vintage buys. This is what creates magic and will come to define your look.

Shopping on the high-street can prove a little challenging because finding the right items takes time – but then again, once you find that one star item, it's so worth it. I like scrolling through store's online shops just to see what's on display. I do most of my shopping online, because most shops offer quick and cheap deliveries. I'm mostly interested in items from brands that come up with their own creative take on things, rather than those who pick and choose from other brands. And I never buy anything without checking out the quality of materials used.

These are my favourite high street shops:

One of my absolute favourites, H&M, doesn't really need an introduction. But I do find their shops a little confusing and unfortunately most of the really budget-friendly offers you find in the shops are rarely available online. So, you have to decide which departments you prefer, as this will help ease your way through the maze. I love their essentials range, because it focuses on materials, shapes and colours. I'm a big fan of their sustainable concept and other initiatives that help preserve the environment. Their Conscious Collection – which puts the focus on sustainable materials and techniques – is looking great. Time and again, I'm surprised by what they manage to create from sustainable materials.

ZARA

ZARA is a must in this category. They are extremely talented when it comes to creating inspiring online look-books and fashion series where they interpret the coming season's trends. Their collections cover everything from completely clean and minimalistic styles to the more colourful and Spanish-inspired styles, which is, after all, the brand's country of origin.

ZARA is also very quality-conscious, and they are frontrunners in terms of combining great shapes with exquisite materials, not least in relation to their accessories. However, it's still a good idea to always check the label describing the materials used, as looks can be deceptive.

This British brand carries a huge range of items inspired by British designs, which are not always compatible with Scandinavian aesthetics. I am fond of their Unique line, which consists of quality styles in neutral or often slightly toned-down colours. Their collaboration with the online store Net-A-Porter, where you can buy select styles from their catwalk collection, is nothing short of awesome!

Topshop

This is H&M's more expensive line, and they truly master the Scandinavian aesthetics. Their prices are higher because they put a bigger focus on quality, and they are known for super cashmere coats and knitwear as well as highly delicate lingerie collections.

COS

This is a British brand whose style universe is very consistent and pure. I actually prefer their men's collection, featuring cardigan blazers, cashmere knitwear and crackling white cotton shirts. Their women's collection is also good, with lots of feminine dresses for special occasions as well as fitted trouser suits.

REISS

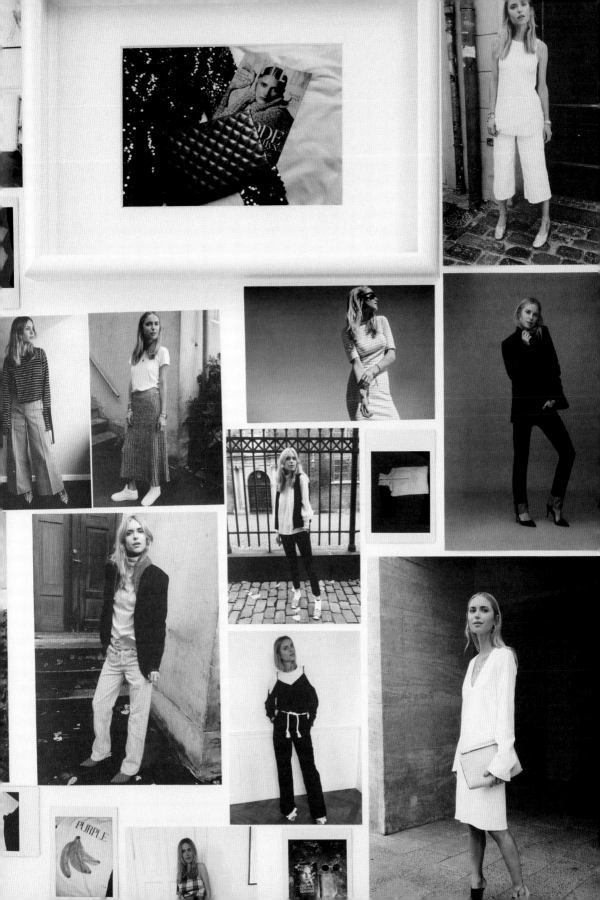

My Top 10

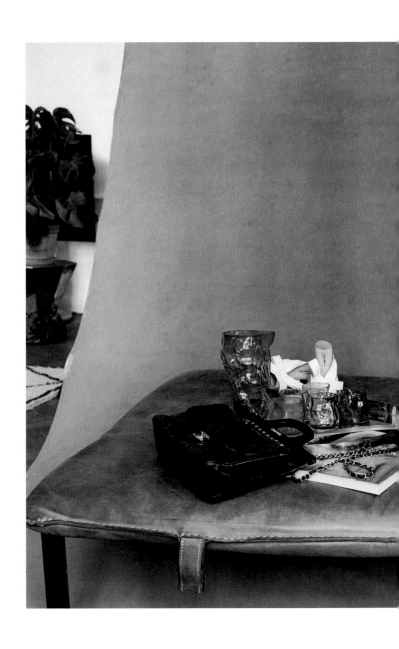

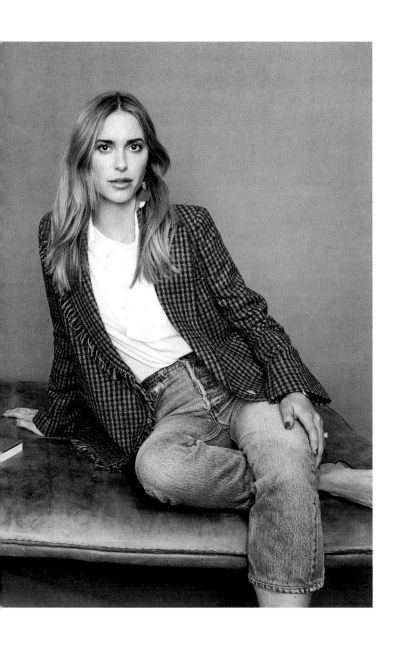

Favourite Scandi Brands

I have a number of go-to Scandinavian brands that I've been very fond of for years. Having worked in the fashion industry for more than 10 years, I've grown up with many of them, and I've seen them truly develop in the most wonderful ways and make their mark on the global scene. I've always supported Scandinavian brands by using their items in shoots or by wearing them myself during fashion weeks. As with everything else, it's all about getting the right mix of international and Scandinavian brands.

My top 10 brands each have an individual Scandinavian take on the classic, clean and modern look – with a slight twist.

Acne Studios

My relationship with Acne Studios is special, not least because I worked in their first Copenhagen-based shop in 2004. Back then, they only sold basic T-shirts and jeans with distinctive red stitching and a flame logo. This brand has taken an impressive turn though, going from being mainly a jeans brand to a proper fashion house. And I'll gladly admit that I feel very proud each time I watch one of their shows at Paris fashion week. A lot of my go-to basic items are from Acne Studio and I wear them till they come apart at the seams.

Agger-Flachs

One of my favourite brands was created by two Danish stylists, Kathrine Agger and Nanna Flachs. Their collections focus on timeless classics rather than passing trends, and you'll find several identical items from one season to the next with only subtle changes in material and colour. What I like about them is their uncompromising stance on quality and fit. I also like the fact that Kathrine and Nanna based their entire concept on favourite items from their personal wardrobes, including a Japanese army-green polo shirt, which is 52 years old. As I write this, they've only been around for six seasons, and yet they've managed to create a sharp, Scandinavian aesthetic that places great value on comfort.

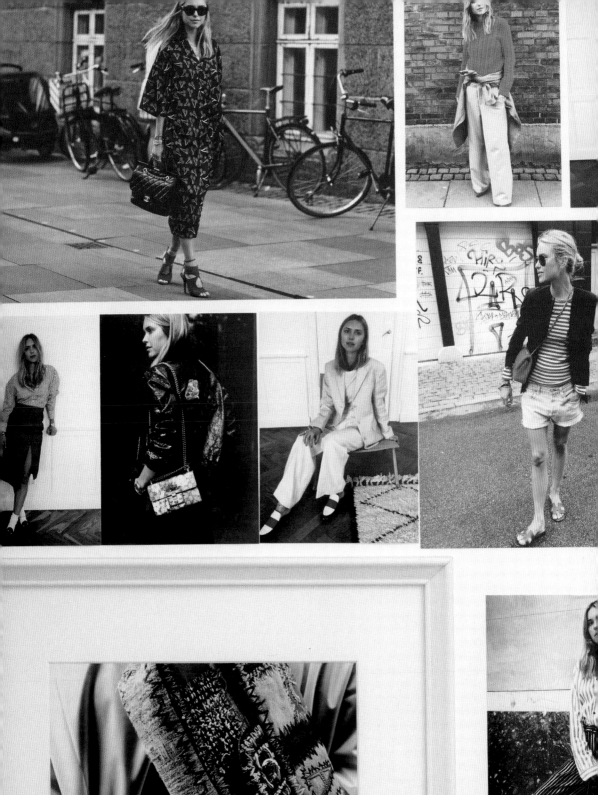
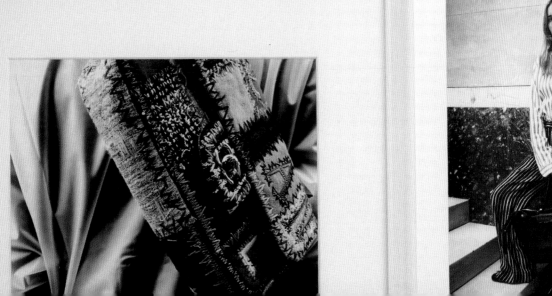

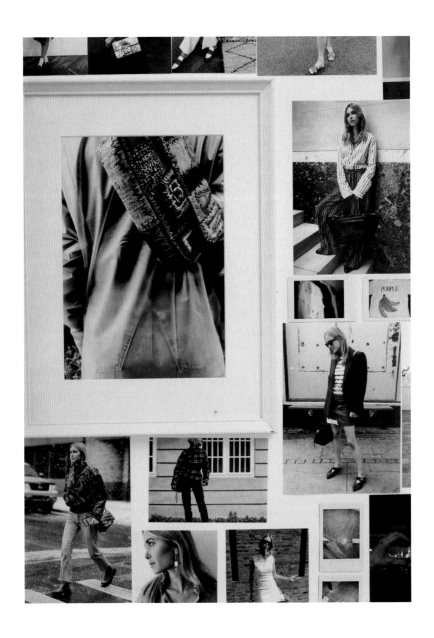

Ganni

In 2007, Head of Design Ditte and her husband Nicolaj Reffstrup bought their way into the company, and since then Ganni has evolved from a small Danish brand to a large international fashion company, selling clothes, shoes, accessories and lingerie. They wanted to create favourites for every woman's wardrobe. And they have succeeded. Their collections embrace everything from pure classics to trend-based styles with a twist.

Filippa K

Filippa Knutsson and Patrik Kihlborg created this Swedish fashion house in 1993, and now their clothes have become an indispensable part of the Scandinavian wardrobe. Filippa K equals timeless designs, simplicity and quality. In my opinion, they manage to create styles that are essential to any wardrobe.

This Danish jeweller is more than 100 years old, and is characterised by its consistent aesthetics, craftsmanship and amazing quality. I've visited their archive – a truly overwhelming and incredibly inspiring experience. Originally, Georg Jensen worked mainly in silver, but these days they're adding more and more gold, which personally I'm very happy about. All my favourite bracelets are from Georg Jensen; especially my chain with diamonds from their Dune collection. This is without a shadow of doubt the one piece of jewellery, aside from my engagement ring, that has received the most compliments.

Georg Jensen

Anne-Dorthe Larsen and Katrine Rabjerg launched Nué Notes in 2007. At the time, they were partners and co-owners of an exclusive shop in Copenhagen. They started with just one leather collection, which quickly became immensely popular. Shortly afterwards, they took advantage of an opportunity to expand their collection adding a number of simple, classic items, including chunky knitwear, shirts and dresses in delicate materials and wonderful colours to wear every day. One of my favourite shirts is by them (the one with the Mandarin collar), and I wear it several times during any week.

Mads Nørgaard is the son of Jørgen, who created the classic, striped top – the famous 101, which has been a regular item in my wardrobe since my early school days. Mads started out as a head designer then, after a few years, he opened his own shop, Strøget, on Copenhagen's pedestrian shopping street. In later years, he has turned out to be highly capable of creating wonderfully feminine and modern high-quality designs in addition to lovely knitwear, often incorporating the legendary stripes you'll find in most of his designs.

It's no coincidence that this Danish jeweller has become immensely popular in just four years. Orit Elhanati's collections definitely reflect her Middle Eastern background, but she somehow manages to combine this with Scandinavian aesthetics in ways that make her designs feel really exciting and unique. The jewellery is minimally treated, and the organic shapes make for extreme exclusivity. When my future husband surprised me with an engagement ring, I was extremely happy (and relieved!) that Orit Elhanati had been involved. She has quite simply designed the most beautiful ring I've ever laid eyes on.

In 2003, Malene Birger established a brand in her own name, which quickly made it onto the international markets. She became known for her highly elegant and glamorous designs, often inspired by earlier fashion icons. Right from the onset, the entire By Malene Birger range was extremely consistent, and in my opinion, it's one of the only genuine fashion houses in Denmark. In 2014, Malene decided to leave her own brand, which meant putting her close design partner, Christina Exsteen, in the driving seat. Christina has already made a huge impact by creating simpler and very usable designs, which are easy to include in your everyday wardrobe.

The Danish jeweller Sophie Bille Brahe has a keen eye for avant-garde designs and modern luxury items, and in 2011, she decided to launch her own brand. She creates elegant, timeless jewellery with a Scandinavian twist and a fresh take on pearls and diamonds. Astronomy is a central source of inspiration, undoubtedly fuelled by her family's passion for observing the sky. Her innovative approach is admirable and she's made her mark internationally, which is why you'll find her in the best shops. I always wear two of her iconic designs; her diamond-studded ear cuff and her delicate double ring, as they upgrade my otherwise casual style significantly.

Sophie Bille Brahe

Sneaking in secretly to 11th place, you'll find a brand that occupies a very special place in my heart, the Danish outerwear brand, Rains. Although it's only three years old, it's already making a huge impact internationally, and currently they're collaborating with Colette and Opening Ceremony among others. In addition to being practical when it rains – which is often in Scandinavia! – their look is truly stylistically consistent, functional and thorough.

Rains

How To
Stay Pretty

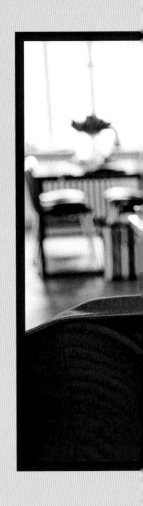

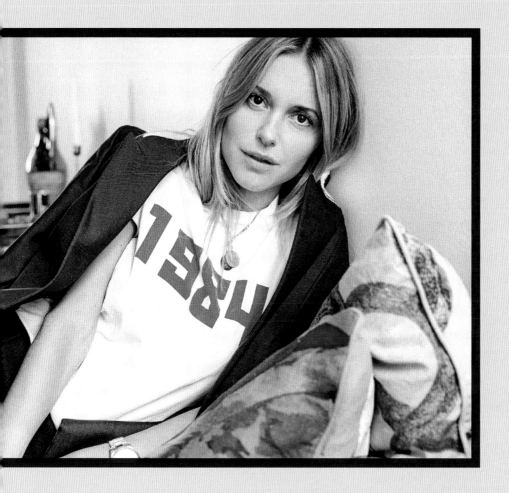

Living In
The Fast Lane

Blonde hair, blue eyes and flawless skin featured in all my childhood drawings of beautiful princesses, and it's also the stereotype of what most people consider a Scandinavian look. Indeed, I know plenty of people who fit the description. Unfortunately, though, I seem to fall slightly outside this category, as I have brown eyes and mousy 'wannabe' blonde hair. I do have delicate and generally healthy skin, although this can be a challenge as our climate swings from very cold winters to semi-warm summers.

I'm not an expert on beauty, and so I cannot speak for others, but I am very knowledgeable about my body and skin and what works for me. That's not to say that I'm closed to suggestions, and I happily invest both time and money in taking proper care of myself.

Most of the products I use are Scandinavian, as we really do lead the field in organic, sustainable beauty products. In Scandinavia, we are very concerned with the environment, particularly when it comes to our food, our skin and our children – and it's something I hope will also influence the entire clothes industry. My products will never be 100 per cent organic, though – I try to use as many organic products as I can, and there is a wide range of quality products available. However, organic nail polish, for example, does not work for me, and so I'll have my shellac nails done once every 3–4 weeks. I love the fun, colourful and eye-catching combinations that create the unexpected contrast in what otherwise is a balanced Scandinavian look.

These are my personal favourite products
from Scandinavian brands:

Organic brands:

— Anti-aging Serum and Facial Oil
  by Rudolph Care
— Radiance Highlighter by Kjær Weiss
— Age-Defence Micellar Water
  by Karmameju
— Exfoliating Algae Hand & Body
  Wash by RAAW in a Jar
— Supreme Moisture Mask by Nuori

Other products:

— Lip Cure and Anti-Aging Molecular
  Messenger Cream by Tromborg
— Dark Spot Fix by Verso
— Pure Nurture Facial Water
  by Ole Henriksen
— Bibliothèque Scented Candle
  by Byredo

My little helpers

I have my regular 'helpers', I call them my life lines because they help me maintain my body once a month and sometimes more. As I'm not that great at looking after my body, I consider it an investment. I've persuaded my four 'helpers', all of whom I've been seeing for years, to share a few tips as well as their take on the Scandinavian look.

Skin

Personally, I really like the natural look without too much make-up (in fact, preferably as little as possible). The focus should be on healthy and well-groomed skin, natural brows and lashes as well as a casual hairdo, which all fits beautifully with the simple aesthetics attributed to the Scandinavian look.

I take skincare very seriously, even more so than I let on, not least because as I grow older I need to pay more attention to my skin. Great skin doesn't need make-up, and you can easily upgrade with a little lipstick in the evening. The same goes for your hair, which in my opinion only becomes increasingly dry and dull the more products you use. That may sound a little boring, but it's not to say that I don't put effort into my natural look. My job means that I constantly find myself on aeroplanes, working all hours of the day, doing shoots that require lots of make-up and hairdos styled with products I would never contemplate using myself. I'm also exposed to numerous changes in climate as well as jetlag, so I have to work really hard if I'm not to break out in all sorts of unpleasantries.

I try to stick to my morning and evening routines. Sometimes I have to skip one or the other, and only rarely are these routines enough on their own to maintain balanced skin. I do have one special routine, which I very rarely skip, and that's a two-minute facial massage morning and evening, which I do while applying some sort of cream or facial oil. I read about it in a magazine once, and I've done it ever since – circular movements around my forehead as well as gentle strokes in sensitive areas, like near my eyes.

For the last six years, I've treated myself to a facial once a month. I make sure I write down each appointment in my diary and try to stick to it, as I know that facials make a huge difference to the overall condition of my skin.

My therapist, Line Friis, specialises in holistic treatments, which means intense work with muscle, tissue and psyche. This approach is very common in Scandinavia. Her expertise lies in reducing lines in a natural way by massage, and I'll recommend her treatments over Botox or other invasive treatments any day. Many of us have quite tense facial muscles, and that creates wrinkles, but after each treatment my skin is always smooth and glowing in a way I unfortunately find it impossible to create myself.

According to Line: 'Scandinavian skin is often characterised by being quite pale and very delicately structured. Scandinavian skin is often very sensitive and only rarely oily. If treated correctly, it can become almost porcelain-perfect.'

Massage your face with high-quality oil when you take a bath. The combination of steam, massage and oil will leave a beautiful glow.

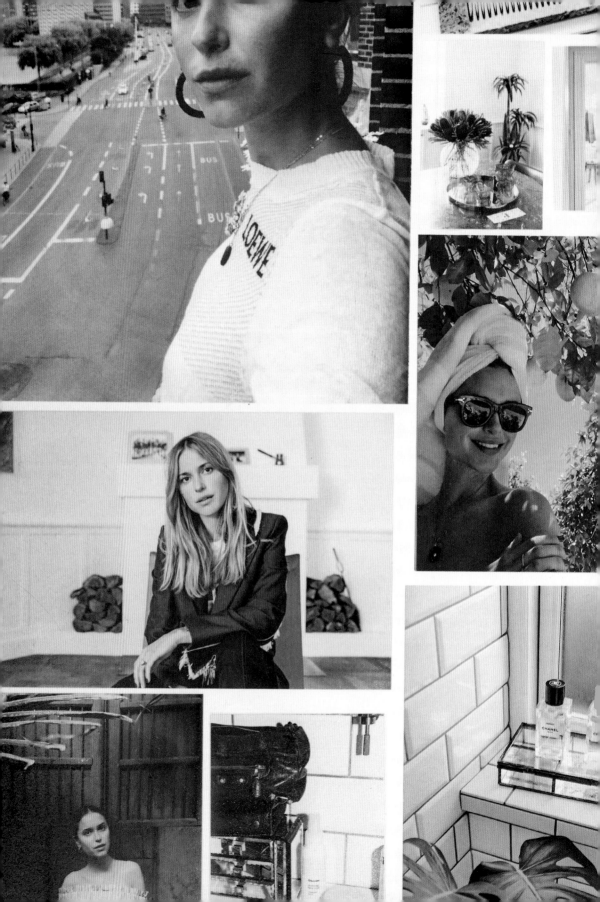

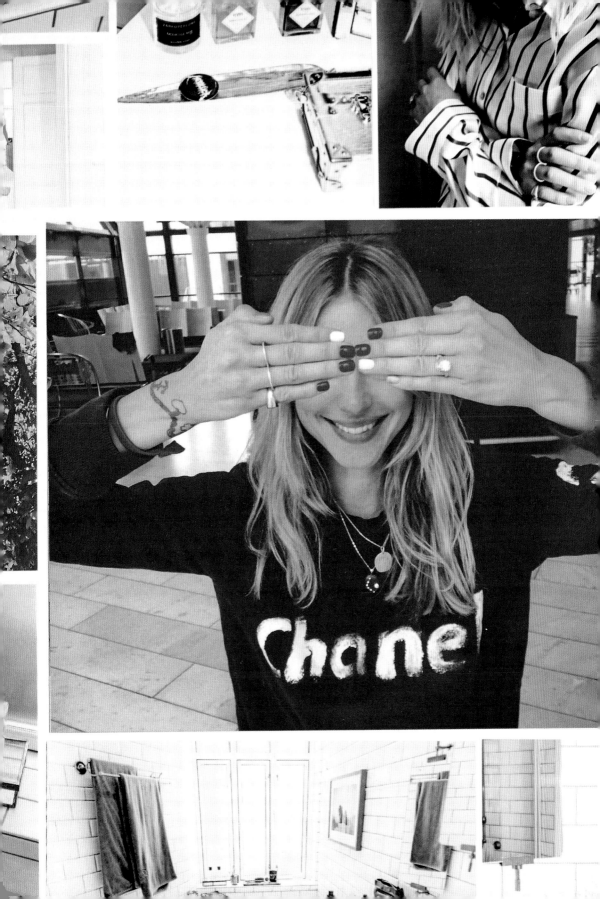

When I look back on some of the haircuts and styles I've subjected myself to, there's quite a level of experimentation – to put it mildly! Up until the age of around 13, my mother cut my hair, which resulted in a classic Playmobil bob – only it would be a little uneven and the fringe would be too short. After that, I let my hair grow long and lovely. Then, one day, someone stopped me in the street and asked if I would like to become a hair model, and so for a short while I didn't have much say in how my hair was cut. I walked out of the salon once with a blonde undercut bob and a black asymmetrical fringe! I cried for weeks, but the damage was already done. So from there on I experimented with everything from black hair à la Cleopatra to curls. However, when I started modelling, I had to stop playing around with my hair so much, as I discovered that the natural look was preferable to most employers.

I often tie my hair in a small knot at the back after washing it, and then I leave it to air-dry, as this adds volume and shine when I loosen it again after a few hours.

To get your hair to look natural and shiny, you need to take good care of it, and you need a really good hairdresser. I was fortunate enough to find one a few years ago. Your hair is affected by the health of your body, as I found out the hard way. During busy times when I do lots of different jobs that include styling my hair on a daily basis, my hair will become lifeless and eventually fall out. It's been excruciatingly frustrating because I wasn't aware of the consequences of driving myself so hard. Time and again, my wonderful hairdresser, Mie Harritz, who's done my hair for five years now, has had to tell me to calm down. Fortunately, she's got to know my hair inside out and she's taught me a lot. After all, hair is so integral to your look. Mie dyes my hair regularly, but she always keeps it natural looking. The downside is no comments from my partner, even when I've spent three-to-four hours at the hairdresser's! But then again, that's how it should be, if you ask me, because I don't want people to notice that my hair is dyed. That's not to say that we Scandinavians never go crazy and try out exotic hair styles, but more often than not, we'll stick with the classic styles, as we know that they work best for us.

Mie Harritz sums it up when she says: 'The typical fashion-conscious Scandinavian woman values a low-key, uncomplicated yet luxurious look.'

Last but not least, it's important to take good care of your body. I try to remember that my body bears the brunt of a lot of stress – whether I'm working in uncomfortable positions on aeroplanes, or functioning with not enough sleep… and so the list continues. In addition to using lovely creams and oils on my skin, I know my body also needs exercise, as well as times of peace and relaxation. I'm a morning person, and I usually start my day with 15 minutes of meditation followed by a run outside. These are two rituals I try to always perform, no matter where in the world I find myself. It clears my head and it makes me feel confident. I try to include other types of exercise, such as yoga or workouts, but finding the time is not always easy.

Over the last few years, Scandinavians have started paying much more attention to our body's wellbeing. We book massages and other types of alternative treatments, and it's definitely become something we prioritise in our everyday lives.

I love alternative treatments, because I always learn something new and occasionally find out facts about my body I wasn't aware of. I think I've probably tried most things now, but the one thing I will always return to is reflexology, because it boosts my immune system, reduces my stress levels and energises me.

According to reflexologist Lisbeth Heckscher: 'Reflexology is a wonderful and recognised treatment, which restores the body's natural balance. Treatments benefit vital organs, the nervous system as well as the lymphoid system. It stimulates overall circulation, improves the transportation of oxygen and thus also the secretion of toxins, and this balances the body.'

Reflexology is a soft, yet effective treatment for many physical illnesses, but it will also boost a tired body suffering the effects of a busy and stressful working life.

Ever since I was a young child, massages were high on the wish list when my group of girlfriends would get together. I was good at doing the other girls' hair, but the return favour would always have to be a massage, and preferably a scalp massage. If I could afford it (and had the time!), I would have a massage every day. As that's not really an option, my wonderful partner has had to suffice, and fortunately, I can sometimes get him to give in and treat my tired shoulders and neck to a massage.

Massage makes your body relax; it improves your mood as well as your sleep, which is important for those of us who lead really busy lives. This is also why I'll gladly allocate 90 minutes for a massage once every month with my regular masseuse Heidi Maltby, who truly understands the body's anatomy and always knows exactly what I need.

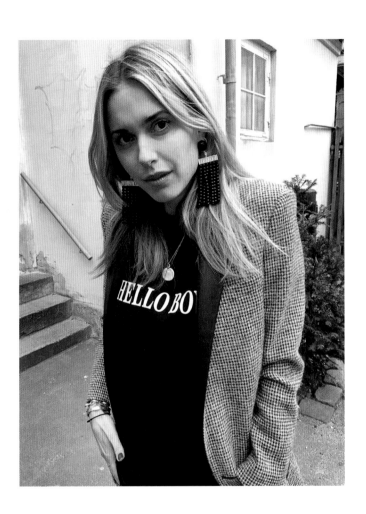

Heidi says: 'Scientific experiments have shown that massage affects our immune system, i.e., you become better at fighting diseases. Those who receive massages regularly fall ill less often, and they fight chronic diseases more successfully. Twenty minutes is enough to lower the level of the stress hormone cortisol, which weakens your immune system.'

Regular massages make us aware of our bodies, which, in turn makes us more susceptible to changes that may imply that something's wrong. This could be tense muscles telling us that we're overworked, or it may be an illness or disease whose symptoms we notice earlier on, before it develops into something serious.

Knowing that I've treated my body and thus myself to something beneficial makes me feel really good about myself. Generally speaking, Scandinavian women are very independent, both in terms of work and private life, which means we tend to deal with lots of issues on our own. So occasionally, we must remember to prioritise ourselves; indulging in quiet moments when nothing is allowed to interrupt, whether that's a walk in the woods, meditation or simply reading a book.

How
to Dress

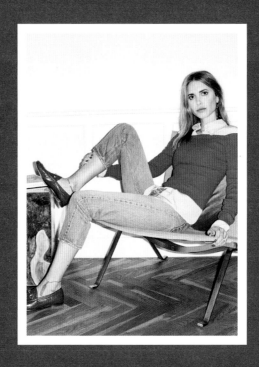

Scandinavian

Those are all the tips I have for now, and I hope I leave you feeling inspired, wiser and ready to create your own Scandinavian look. Even though clothes belong in the category of material goods, they are still hugely important in creating and expressing your personal look. Dressing Scandinavian is a question of balancing style and emotion while emphasising confidence and contentedness.

If you've not started the shopping list for your Scandinavian wardrobe yet, below you'll find a very short summary of what to look for:

Blazer

Jeans

Colourful high heels

Striped top

Jewellery

A quality handbag

Shirts

Index

Acknowledge

I'm so pleased to have the opportunity to thank you all – those of you who made it this far. Thank you!

Thank you to my right-hand woman and second half of my brain, Rikke Charlotte Larsen. You are so incredibly tough and a great gift in my life – without you, there would be so many spelling mistakes, there'd be no photos and I would have spent way too many evenings alone in my office.

Thank you to my partner, agent and best friend, Hannah Løffler, who constantly interrupted my sacred writing sessions, either by way of long phone conversations or by presenting job offers that seriously challenged my writing process! There are so many things I should thank you for, because you've made my work and my everyday life so much more fun and meaningful. I have no doubt that we'll stay glued together for as long as we live.

Without the two of you this book would not have seen the light of day.

ments

Thank you Lars Dyhr, LOW – you are a graphic design genius and a good friend. I'm so grateful for your work, your creative sparring, as well as the visual and graphic results, which I would never have reached had you not helped me.

Thank you Marianne Kiertzner and People's Press, who contacted me one summer's day and suggested that I should write a book on style, which I'd in fact been contemplating only a few months earlier. Thank you for believing in me and my crazy ideas and expensive aesthetic suggestions.

Thank you to my family and friends, who have been a constant and never-ending source of inspiration and support.

To the man in my life, who is so incredibly patient, encouraging and creative, and who spoiled me with goodies during long nights of writing, and who is the best sparring partner ever. I love you!

Thank you to my family of street-photographers worldwide – you've lifted my career and contributed immensely to my former blog and now this book. Thank you for always catching me at the right moment – without a camel toe, and never tripping over the curb.

Finally, a huge thank you to all my readers, who continue to follow me on social media.